AF712774

# Neurology

## Made Ridiculously Simple

Stephen Goldberg, MD
Professor Emeritus
University of Miami
Miller School of Medicine
Miami FL

Damon R. Salzman, MD
Department of Neurology
Broward Health Physician Group
Fort Lauderdale FL

MEDMASTER

Copyright © 2026 by Medmaster, Inc.

All rights reserved. This book is protected by copyright. No part of it may be reproduced, stored in a retrieval system, or transmitted in any form or by any means (electronic, mechanical, photocopying, recording or otherwise) without written permission from the copyright owner.

ISBN #978-1-962445-10-8
eISBN #978-1-962445-11-5

*Made in the United States of America*

Published by Medmaster, Inc.

Cover by Jordan Collver and Owen Watts

# Works by Stephen Goldberg

**Books:**
Clinical Neuroanatomy Made Ridiculously Simple
The Four-Minute Neurologic Exam
Goldberg's Brain Model
Ophthalmology Made Ridiculously Simple
Jonah: The Anatomy of the Soul
The Jonah Principle: The Basis for Human and Machine Consciousness
Consciousness, Information, and Meaning: The Origin of the Mind
Consciousness: How the Mind Arises from the Brain
Anatomy of the Soul: Mind, God, and the Afterlife
Consciousness Made Ridiculously Simple
Is the Mind Immortal?: The Origin of Consciousness
Clinical Anatomy Made Ridiculously Simple
Clinical Physiology Made Ridiculously Simple
Clinical Biochemistry Made Ridiculously Simple
Clinical Genetics Made Ridiculously Simple
Clinical Biostatistics and Epidemiology Made Ridiculously Simple
LiveCode Lite: Computer Programming Made Ridiculously Simple
Clinical Hematology Made Ridiculously Simple
War Against the Germs: Epidemics, Microorganisms, and Biowarfare
Med'Toons
Endocrinology Made Ridiculously Simple
Gastroenterology Made Ridiculously Simple
Neurology Made Ridiculously Simple

**Computer Programs:**
Neurologic Localization
Atlas of Ophthalmology
Atlas of Microbiology
Atlas of Human Diseases
Differential Diagnosis
Atlas of Dermatology
Atlas of Orthopedics
Medsearcher

# About the Authors

Stephen Goldberg, M.D., a graduate of the Albert Einstein College of Medicine, is a physician, researcher, teacher, computer programmer, writer, and musician/composer. Dr. Goldberg has published numerous medical and scientific papers on neuronal development and regeneration through research at the Albert Einstein College of Medicine, National Institutes of Health, New York Medical College and the University of Miami Miller School of Medicine. He practiced Neurology, Ophthalmology, and Family Medicine at various times in his career, with Board certification in the latter two fields. He is a past medical director of the National Parkinson Institute and present Professor Emeritus at the University of Miami Miller School of Medicine, where he taught neuroanatomy for 25 years. Dr. Goldberg has authored many books in a diversity of medical/scientific areas, including the best-selling *Clinical Neuroanatomy Made Ridiculously Simple*; books on Consciousness; Gross Anatomy; Physiology; Biochemistry; Genetics; Biostatistics and Epidemiology; Ophthalmology; Hematology; Microbiology; Endocrinology; Gastroenterology; and Computer Programming, as well as many interactive computer programs on various medical topics, including *Neurologic Localization*. His reputation is that of an educator who can simplify complex topics. He received the George Paff Most Outstanding Professor Teaching Award 11 times at the U of M and was invited in 2004 to be the keynote speaker at the medical school graduation commencement at the Washington University School of Medicine in St. Louis for his work in medical education. He is a past president of the Medmaster Publishing Company, where he is currently Editor-in-Chief.

Dr. Damon Salzman is a board-certified neurologist and sleep medicine specialist with over two decades of clinical and academic experience. He earned his medical degree from Northwestern University Medical School and completed his neurology residency and sleep disorders fellowship at Harvard Medical School/Beth Israel Deaconess Medical Center.

Dr. Salzman previously served as Director of the Sleep-Wake Disorders Center at New York-Presbyterian Hospital and Weill Cornell Medical College, and later as Director of the

Florida Lou Ruvo Center of Brain Health at Cleveland Clinic Florida, where he directed the behavioral neurology and memory disorders program. He also served as a neurologist for the NFL's Chronic Traumatic Encephalopathy program. Currently, he practices at Broward Health, where he serves as core teaching faculty for the neurology residency program.

His academic background includes a Master of Studies from Oxford University's Centre for Postgraduate Hebrew Studies, reflecting his scholarly interests beyond medicine. Dr. Salzman has authored numerous publications on neurological disorders and has been recognized as one of the Top Doctors by Castle Connolly.

Dr. Salzman lives in South Florida with his wife and three children.

# Preface

This book is for medical, nursing, and PA students, primary care physicians, and other health professionals to provide a general overview of neurology. Neurology can be so complex that it becomes difficult to gain an overall picture of the numerous neurological pathways, intricate exam methods, diseases, and treatments. The book tries to present clinical neurology in a way that enables the reader to quickly grasp the subject by emphasizing its most important features, in a way that promotes understanding rather than rote memorization. The clinical focus is on diseases that are more probable, more serious if missed, and more likely to lead to an effective remedy. Chapters on neurologic diseases can be organized according to nervous system *location* (e.g., cerebrum, brain stem, spinal cord, peripheral nerves), according to *disease process* (e.g., infectious, vascular, autoimmune, degenerative, etc.), or according to the way the patient presents to the physician (e.g., weakness, sensory loss, pain, seizure, dizziness, balance problems, memory loss, etc.). We have chosen the latter symptomatic approach, since it is how the patient presents and the immediate practical route to the diagnosis and treatment.

A number of neuroanatomical illustrations are taken from SG's book *Clinical Neuroanatomy Made Ridiculously Simple*, with one important difference. The organization of the brainstem has been simplified, including only that information necessary to determine whether a lesion lies in the brain stem and whether it is in the medulla, pons, or midbrain. Once the examiner knows this, neurologic imaging can determine the precise location and often the pathology. Readers interested in greater detail can find it in *Clinical Neuroanatomy MRS* or in its interactive program *Neurologic Localization*, which is available as a download from the Medmaster website, *www.medmaster.net*.

Any humor in the book is not intended as disrespect for patients or original investigators; it is employed as an educational device to facilitate learning and memory.

Thanks to Phyllis Goldenberg for her excellent proofreading and advice. Dermatology photos are courtesy of Aviva Hopkins Wolgin, M.D. and the American College of Rheumatology.

# Contents

## Part II. Neurologic History, Exam, And Treatment

## Part III. Neurologic Presentations

# PART I. Neuroanatomy Review

The human nervous system has an estimated 86 billion nerve cells (neurons) and a quadrillion nerve cell connections (synapses), give or take a synapse or two. This cell collection can be affected by numerous neurologic diseases with presenting symptoms that commonly include:

- Headache
- Back and Other Pain
- Weakness
- Dizziness and Vertigo
- Numbness or Tingling
- Seizures
- Abnormal Movements
- Balance and Coordination Problems
- Changes in Vision
- Memory Loss or Cognitive Decline
- Speech and Language Problems
- Changes in Mood or Behavior
- Sleep Disorders

Fortunately, the neurologist has many tools to effectively diagnose and treat them:

- The History
- The Physical Exam
- Imaging
- Spinal Fluid, Blood, and Other Lab Tests
- Pharmacologic and Non-pharmacologic Treatments

Neurologic diseases can affect any area of the nervous system. Key questions the neurologist initially asks about the presenting problem are "**Where** is it located? Is there one location that can account for all the symptoms?" and then, "**What** is it?" which generally falls into one of the categories of the diagnostic mnemonic **VINDICATE ME**:

**V**ascular
**I**nflammatory / Infectious
**N**eoplastic
**D**egenerative
**I**ntoxication or drug withdrawal
**C**ongenital
**A**llergic / Autoimmune
**T**raumatic
**E**ndocrine

**M**etabolic
**E**motional

Other immediate considerations: How? and Who?:

How urgent is it?: (Emergency vs can wait)
Who should see it?: (Neurology, neurosurgery, ophthalmology, etc.)

Now you don't want to randomly CAT-scan the entire body to find where the problem is, incurring false positives along the way, when it is often possible to precisely pinpoint the disease location, sometimes within millimeters, from the history and physical exam alone. Then, focus on that particular area with imaging, or other tests if needed, to narrow the diagnosis and decide on appropriate therapy. For that reason, it is important to have a basic understanding of the anatomy of the nervous system, as well as a basic technique of the neurologic history and exam. Then you can proceed to neurologic imaging or other tests, if indicated, to make the diagnosis, followed by treatment.

# 1

# *General Organization*

The central nervous system (CNS) includes the cerebrum, cerebellum, brain stem, and spinal cord (**Fig. 1-1**) plus a few scary-sounding structures situated between the brain stem and cerebrum; namely, the *diencephalon* (which includes everything with the name "thalamus"; i.e., the thalamus, hypothalamus, epithalamus and subthalamus) and the *basal ganglia* (which includes the caudate nucleus, the globus pallidus, the putamen, claustrum, and amygdala). Fortunately, it is clinically unimportant to have a detailed understanding of the connections of the diencephalon and basal ganglia. Also, despite the myriad synapses in the central nervous system, there is only one that it is clinically important to know (the connection between upper and lower motor neurons). You'll see why later.

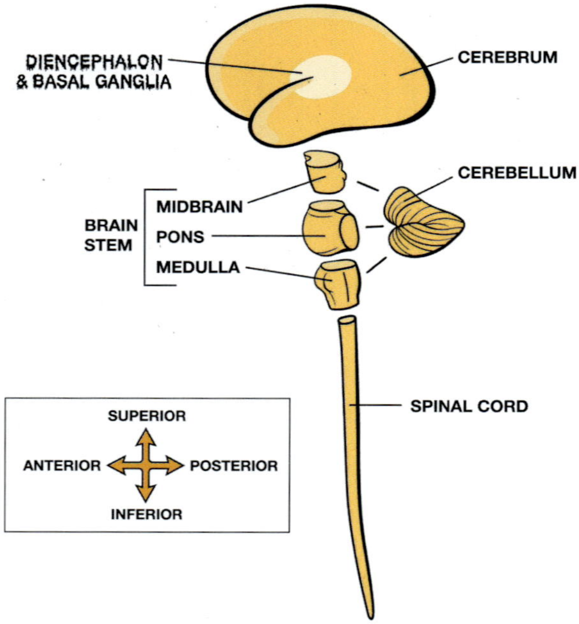


***Figure 1-1*** *The central nervous system. Within the brain stem and spinal cord, the superior-inferior axis is synonymous with the "rostral-caudal" axis, and the anterior-posterior axis is synonymous with the "ventral-dorsal" axis.*

The basic functional unit in the CNS is the neuron (**Fig. 1-2**). Electrophysiological impulses travel down a neuron from its dendrites to the cell body and axon. Information then is chemically transmitted to other neurons via connections known as **synapses**. A chain of such communicating neurons is called a **pathway**. Within the CNS, a bundle of pathway axons is called **a tract, fasciculus, peduncle**, or **lemniscus**. Outside the CNS (i.e., in the peripheral nerves, which connect the CNS with the skin, muscles, and other organ systems), bundles of axons are called **nerves**. So you can immediately see the problem with neuroanatomy. There are too many names for the same thing. But the basic logic of neuroanatomy is simple. We shall try to restrict names to a minimum.

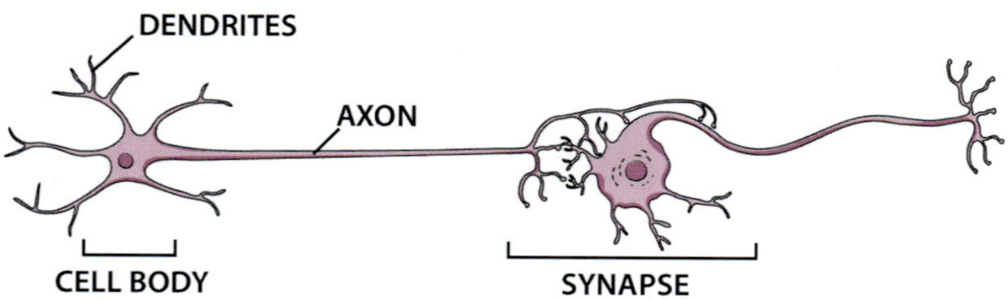


***Figure 1-2*** *The neuron.*

There are 31 pairs of spinal nerves and 12 pairs of cranial nerves. Note that the spinal cord is shorter than the vertebral column so that the spinal nerve roots extend caudally when leaving the spinal cord. This disparity increases at more caudal levels of the cord. The spinal cord ends at about vertebral level L2 but nerves L2-S5 continue caudally as the cauda equina ("horse's tail") to exit by their corresponding vertebrae (**Fig. 1-3**).

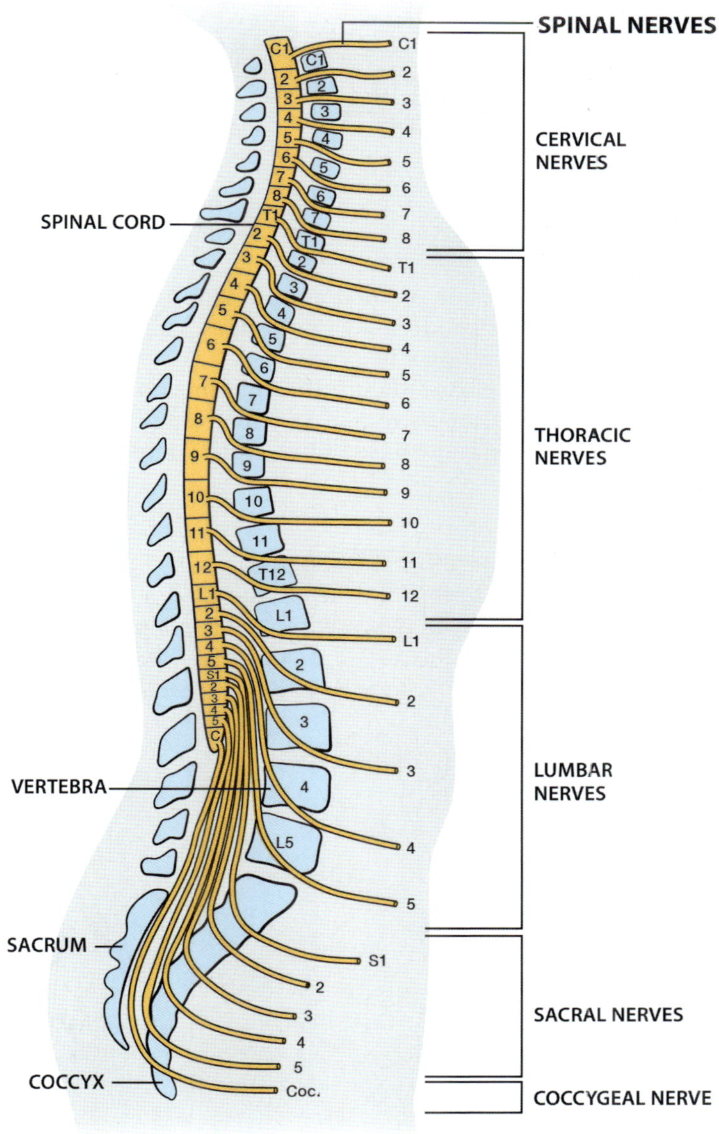


***Figure 1-3*** *The spinal nerves. C, cervical; T, thoracic; L, lumbar; S, sacral; Coc., coccygeal nerve.*

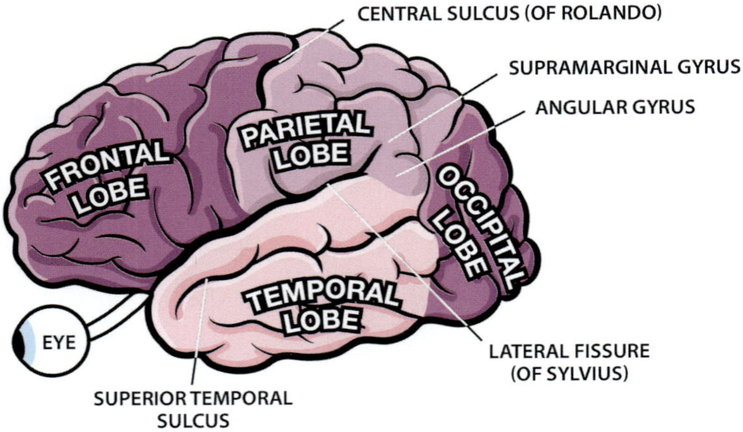


***Figure 1-4*** *The cerebrum.*

Figure 1-4 illustrates the subdivision of the cerebrum into frontal, parietal, occipital and temporal lobes. These are further subdivided into bulges, called **gyri**, and indentations called **sulci** and **fissures** (small and large, respectively).

The brain stem contains three parts—the **midbrain**, **pons** and **medulla** (**Fig. 1-1**). The pons lies squashed against the **clivus**, a region of bone resembling a slide that extends to the foramen magnum, the hole at the base of the skull where the spinal cord becomes the brain stem (**Fig. 1-5**).

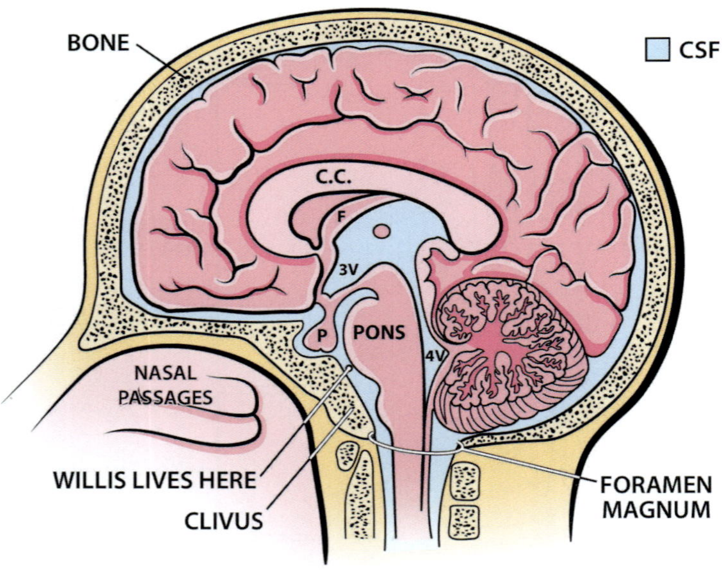


***Figure 1-5*** *Sagittal view of the brain. C.C., corpus callosum—the major connection between the two cerebral hemispheres; f, fornix; 3v, third ventricle; p, pituitary gland; 4v, fourth ventricle. Blue-shaded areas are zones containing cerebrospinal fluid.*

Sometimes the brain stem does "slide down" the clivus, herniating into the foramen magnum. This is a serious clinical condition, generally resulting from a pressure differential between cranial and spinal cavities. Many clinicians therefore are wary in removing cerebrospinal fluid during a spinal tap in patients with high intracranial pressure.

Note the proximity of the clivus to the nasal passages. Sometimes rare invasive tumors of the nasal passages erode and break through the clivus and damage the brain stem. Pituitary tumors may be reached surgically via the nasal passages by producing a hole in the sphenoidal bone, which houses the pituitary gland—the "transsphenoidal approach."

A spider named Willis lives on the pons and its nose fits into the pituitary fossa, but more of this later.

# 2

# Blood Supply, Meninges, and Spinal Fluid

Two main pairs of arteries supply the brain—the two internal carotid arteries and the two vertebral arteries. The vertebral artery changes its name. It's called the basilar artery at the level of the pons and the posterior cerebral artery (PCA) at the level of the cerebrum (**Fig. 2-1**). You'll see why when we discuss Willis, the spider.

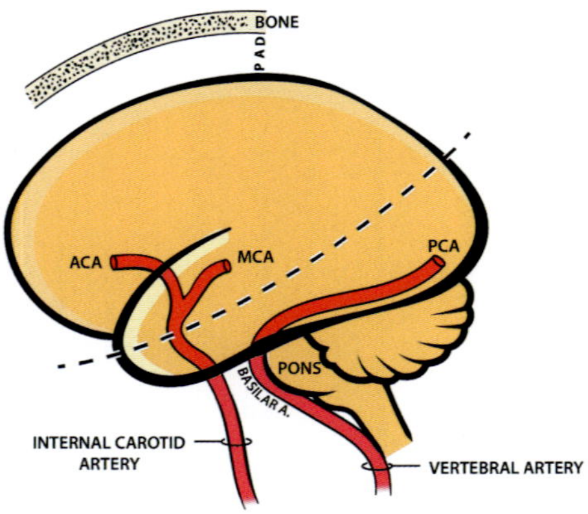


***Figure 2-1*** *The major arterial supply to the brain. ACA, anterior cerebral artery; MCA, middle cerebral artery; PCA, posterior cerebral artery; PAD, pia, arachnoid, dura.*

Note the important imaginary dotted line in **Figure 2-1.** It divides the cerebrum into a front (anterior) and a back (posterior) area. The internal carotid artery supplies the front area. Obstruction of the right carotid artery causes weakness and loss of sensation on the left side of the body (one side of the brain connects with the opposite side of the body). Blockage of the circulation under the dotted line (vertebral artery distribution) affects the circulation to the visual area of the cerebrum, the brain stem, and the cerebellum and may result in visual loss, dizziness, and other problems.

The internal carotid artery divides into an anterior and middle cerebral artery (**Fig. 2-1**). Note (**Fig. 2-2**) that the posterior cerebral artery occupies the entire cerebrum below the dotted line. The middle cerebral artery, though, occupies only the lateral surface of the cerebrum above the dotted line, whereas the anterior cerebral artery occupies the entire midline area of the cerebral hemisphere above the dotted line.

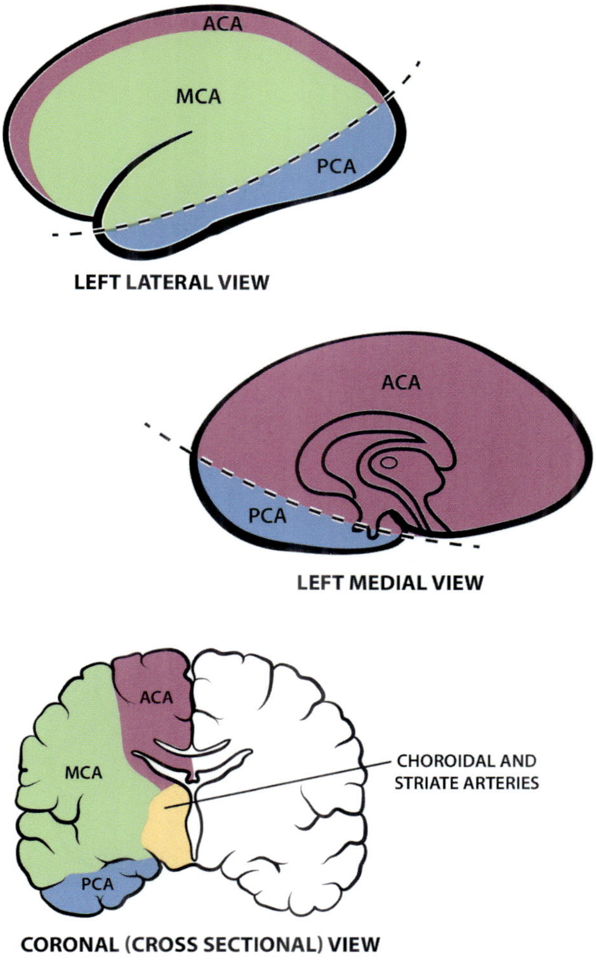


*Figure 2-2* *The cerebral blood circulation. MCA, middle cerebral artery; ACA, anterior cerebral artery; PCA, posterior cerebral artery.*

The brain contains an upside-down man named HAL (H-head, A-arm, L-leg), functionally represented on the cerebral cortex. HAL's lower extremity bends over the top of the cerebrum (**Fig. 2-3**). Therefore, an occlusion of the anterior cerebral artery results in loss of strength and sensation in the lower part of the (opposite) body, whereas an occlusion of the middle cerebral artery predominantly affects strength and sensation in the upper regions of the (opposite) body.

A ferocious spider lives in the brain. His name is Willis! Note (**Figs. 2-4** and **2-5**) that he has a nose, angry eyebrows, two suckers, eyes, a crew cut, antennae, a fuzzy beard), 8 legs, a belly that, according to your point of view, is either thin (basilar artery) or fat (the pons, which lies from one end of the basilar artery to the other), two feelers on his rear legs, and male genitalia. The names in **Figure 2-4** look like those in **Figure 2-1** because they *are* the same structures, seen from different angles. In **Figure 2-4** the brain is seen from below, so the carotid arteries are seen in cross section (Willis' eyes). **Figure 2-4** also explains why the vertebral artery changes its name twice. At first, the two vertebral arteries fuse to form one basilar artery. The basilar artery then divides again into two posterior cerebral arteries.

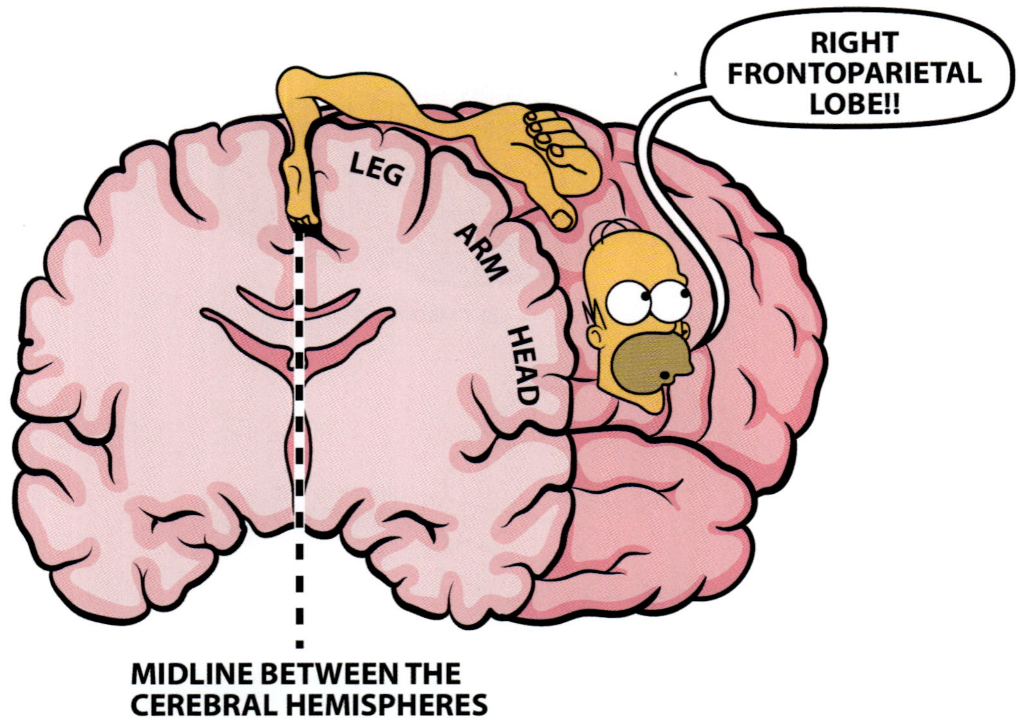


***Figure 2-3** The homunculus.*

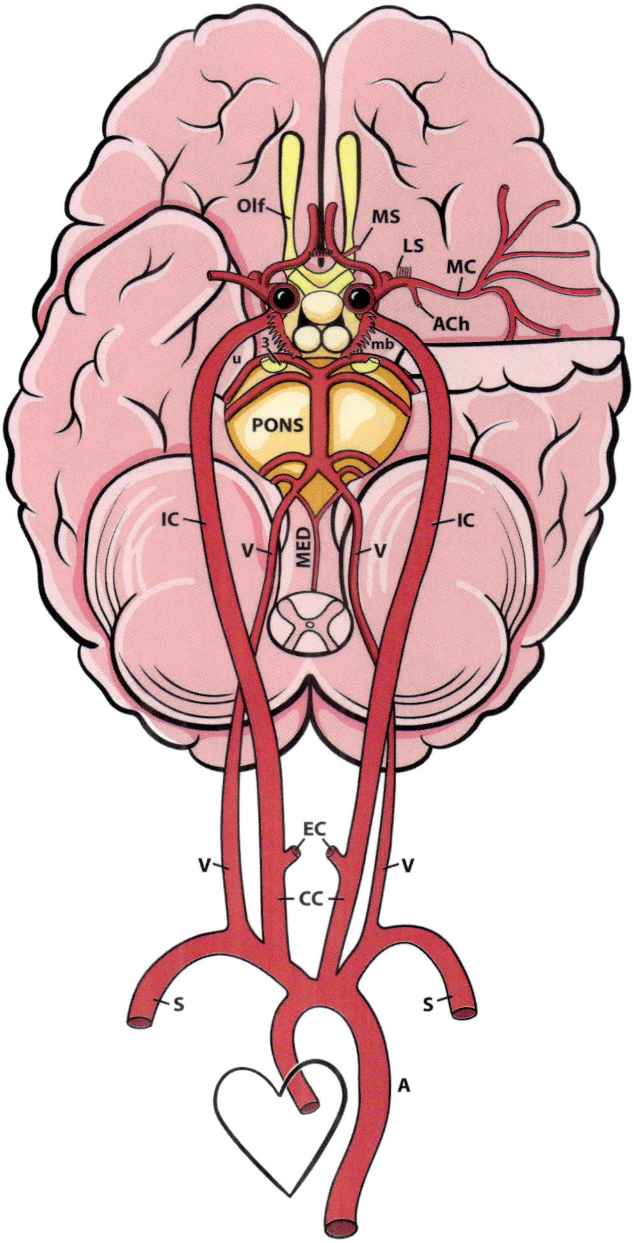


***Figure 2-4*** *The origin of the intracranial arteries from the aorta. Olf., olfactory tract; MS, medial striate artery; LS, lateral striate artery; ACh., anterior choroidal artery; MC, middle cerebral artery; 3, cranial nerve 3; mb, midbrain; u, uncus; IC, internal carotid artery; V, vertebral artery; MED, medulla; EC, external carotid artery; CC, common carotid artery; S, subclavian artery; A, aorta.*

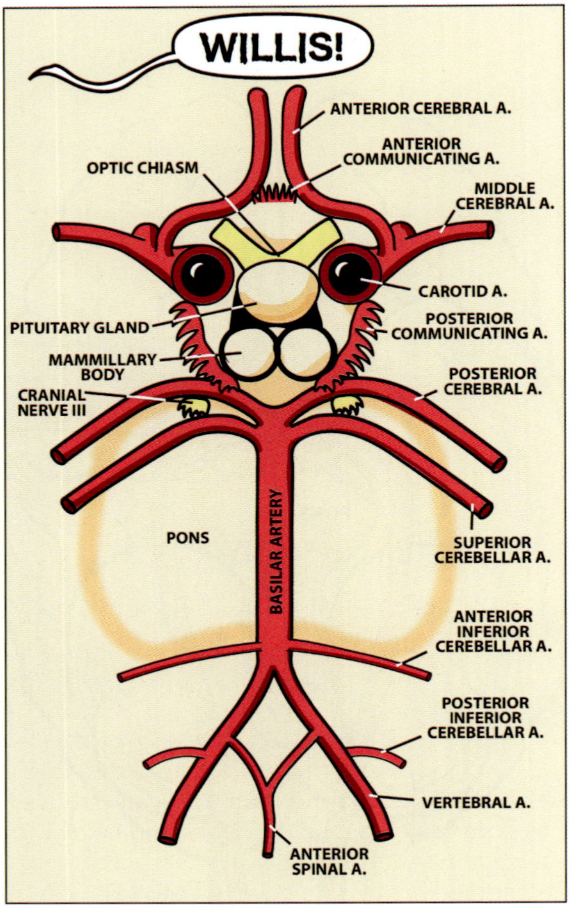


***Figure 2-5*** *Willis!*

An occlusion of the basilar artery at the junction of the two posterior cerebral arteries may result in total blindness, as the posterior cerebral arteries supply the visual cortex. Occlusion of a vertebral artery may result in little or no deficit because of the remaining blood supply from the opposite vertebral artery.

The cerebellar arteries also supply part of the brain stem at their level. The anterior spinal artery supplies the anterior part of the medulla and spinal cord (**Fig. 2-4**). There are also two posterior spinal arteries (not shown), which come off either the vertebral artery or the posterior cerebellar artery. They supply the posterior part of the spinal cord.

The "fuzziness" of the communicating arteries is the ambiguity as to which way blood flows in these vessels. Blood flow in the anterior and posterior communicating arteries (**Fig. 2-5**) shows no particular tendency to go one way or the other. This is logical since blood normally flows up both the carotid and vertebral arteries, equalizing their pressure against one another. Hence, contrast material injected into the right carotid artery generally will not cross over to the left side of the brain via the anterior communicating artery or flow back into the basilar artery across the posterior communicating artery. This all goes to show that the brain is smart. If one of the major vessels is occluded, the communicating arteries function as anastomoses.

Willis has hairy armpits—the third cranial nerve exits between the posterior cerebral artery and the superior cerebellar artery. An aneurysm (a weakness and focal ballooning out of the wall of a blood vessel) which affects either of the above two blood vessels may press upon and damage the third nerve.

There are an anterior, middle, and posterior cerebral artery. It would have been nice to have an anterior, middle, and posterior cerebellar artery, too, but someone inconsiderately named these three arteries differently.

It could have been worse. He could have named them after himself—actually, he did, for he was a real SAP (S-superior cerebellar artery, A-anterior inferior cerebellar artery, P-posterior inferior cerebellar artery). The cerebellar arteries supply not only the cerebellum but also parts of the brain stem. Their occlusion will result in damage to corresponding areas of the brain stem.

## The Veins

Unlike other arteries of the body which have corresponding veins running alongside them, Willis has no female counterpart. This is because he is so ugly that the veins flee in the opposite direction, jumping clear out of the brain and directly into **the dural sinuses** (**Fig. 2-6**). You see, the brain is separated from the cranial bone by a PAD (P-pia, A-arachnoid, D-dura membranes—**Fig. 2-1**), otherwise known as the **meninges**. The pia is thin and vascular (Willis lives in it) and hugs the brain, extending into all its fissures and sulci. The arachnoid lies between the pia and dura, is arachnoid-like, like a gossamer spider web, and avascular. The dura lies up against the bone and is thick and durable, containing a double layer of connective tissue (the outer layer representing periosteum) with thick venous channels, called sinuses, which lie between the two layers. The dura dips down in between the cerebral hemispheres as the **falx cerebri** and in between the cerebrum and cerebellum as the **tentorium cerebelli**. The "PAD" surrounds the entire central nervous system, including the spinal cord and optic nerve.

The term "supratentorial" has been applied notoriously in a clinical sense, to imply that a patient's problem is psychological, and not physiologic. I.e., "His abdominal pain is supratentorial," above the tentorium, "in his head," and not in the abdomen where the pain is reported.

Three main sinuses (**Fig. 2-6**) deserve mention: 1) Spinal fluid drains into the **superior sagittal sinus**. 2) The **cavernous sinus**, into which venous blood drains from the eye, provides a potential source of entry into the brain of orbital and facial infections. Many important structures run by or through the cavernous sinus, including the carotid artery and all the nerves entering the orbit. These can be damaged by disease in this critical area. Sometimes the carotid artery breaks open into the cavernous sinus (a "fistula") resulting in blood backing up into the orbital veins and a protruding eye with dilated blood vessels. 3) The **transverse sinus** runs by the ear and may become involved in inner ear infections (**Fig. 2-6**).

The veins of the brain drain into the **internal jugular vein**, a structure you know well from vampire movies.

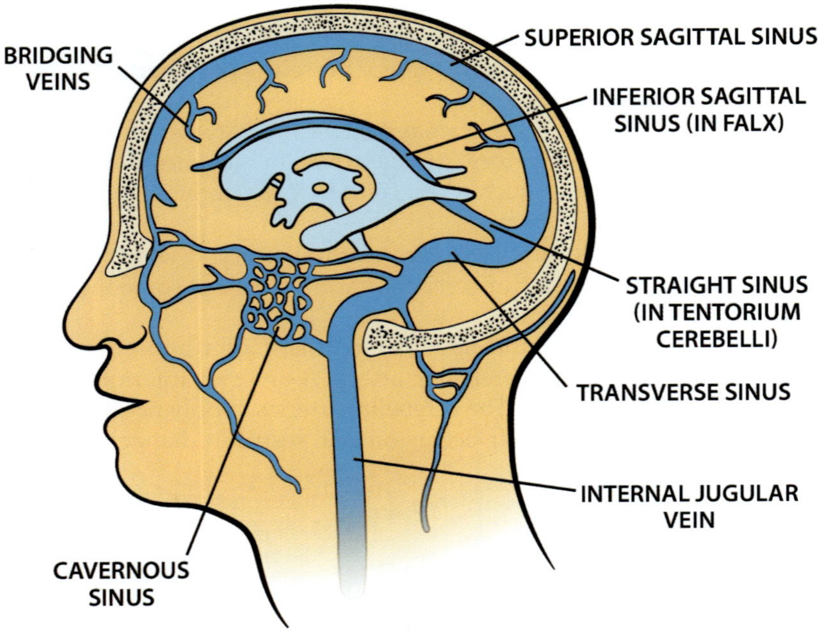


***Figure 2-6*** *The major venous circulation of the brain.*

## The Cerebrospinal Fluid

The brain and spinal cord are hollow—which is fortunate for that means there is less to know (**Fig. 2-7**). Various points in this fluid-filled hollow tube are expanded and termed **ventricles**. The walls of each ventricle contain a specialized structure called the **choroid plexus** which secretes the clear, colorless cerebrospinal fluid (CSF). CSF flows from the two **lateral ventricles** through the two **interventricular foramina** (holes), first into the single mid-line **third ventricle**, from there through the single midline **aqueduct of Sylvius**, next into the single midline **fourth ventricle**, and then passes outside the brain via three openings in the fourth ventricle: a *M*iddle **foramen of *M*agendie** and two *L*ateral **foramina of *L*uschka.** Once outside the brain stem, the CSF enters the subarachnoid space (the space between the arachnoid and pia) and exits into the superior sagittal sinus via specialized structures in the sinus wall called **arachnoid villi**. An obstruction at any point along this pathway will lead to dilation (expansion) of the lateral ventricles, termed *hydrocephalus*. Hydrocephalus from an obstruction outside the brain stem is termed "**communicating hydrocephalus**" since the ventricular system can still communicate with the space outside the nervous system. A CSF obstruction inside the brain or brain stem is termed "**non-communicating" hydrocephalus**, since the ventricular system then cannot communicate with the outside space.

Normally, CSF does not circulate in the central spinal canal of adults as the canal is closed off in places.

Expanded areas of the subarachnoid space are called **cisterns**, the largest of which is the lumbar cistern, between vertebrae L2 (where the spinal cord ends) and S2 (**Fig. 2-7**) in adults. Spinal fluid is extracted from this space during the "spinal tap" (lumbar puncture). Do not panic on doing a spinal tap. There is plenty of room, some five vertebral interspaces, and the crest of the iliac bone provides a landmark to determine approximately the center of the lumbar cistern. There is little chance of hitting the spinal cord and it is uncommon to damage the spinal roots of the cauda equina. In newborns, the anatomy differs, the spinal cord ending (*conus medullaris*) at about vertebra L3 rather than the adult level of L1 or L2, ascending as the child grows. Normal CSF opening pressure is 6-25 cm H20 in adults.

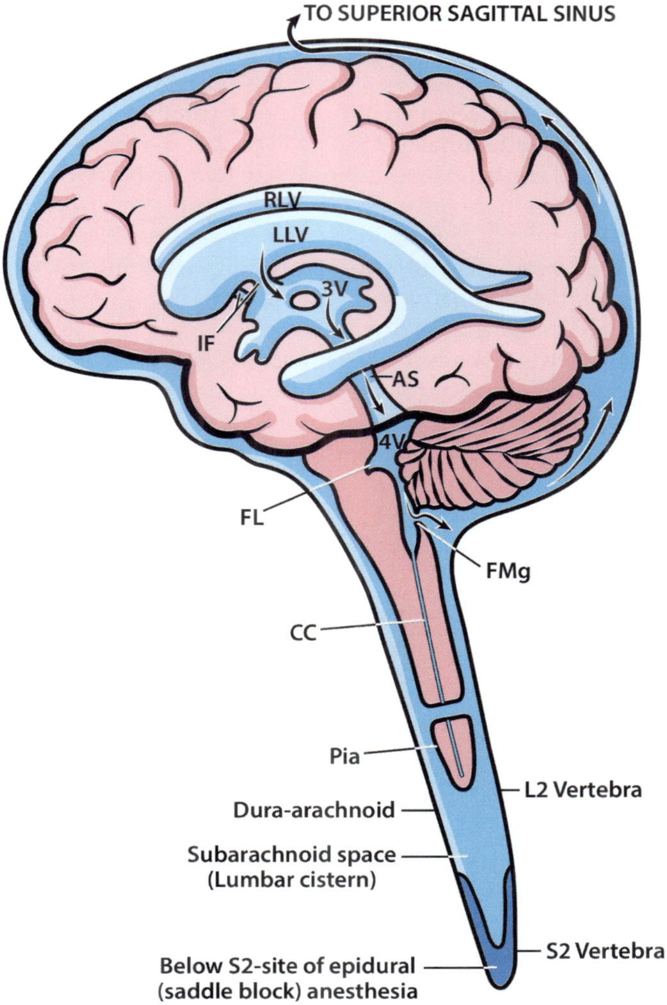


***Figure 2-7*** *The cerebrospinal fluid (CSF) circulation. Arrows indicate the direction of flow of CSF. RLV, right lateral ventricle, LLV, left lateral ventricle; 3V, third ventricle; IF, inter-ventricular foramina; AS, aqueduct of Sylvius; 4V, fourth ventricle; FL, foramen of Luschka, FMg, foramen of Magendie, CC, central canal.*

The CSF flows freely throughout the subarachnoid space; thus, a subarachnoid hemorrhage, usually the result of leakage from an aneurysm in the region of Willis, is felt as a severe neckache or backache, reflecting the seepage of blood down to spinal cord regions. A spinal tap will reveal such bleeding. Symptoms in meningitis are similar, because of the diffusion of pus cells down the subarachnoid space.

A **subdural hemorrhage** results from tearing the bridging veins (**Fig. 2-6**) that connect the brain and dural sinuses. In an **epidural hemorrhage**, blood collects between the dura and bone, the result of tearing arteries, particularly the **middle meningeal artery** which lies outside the dura and forms a groove in the cranial bone. Epidural hemorrhage generally coincides with a skull fracture. Large subdural and epidural hemorrhages can compress the brain and cause significant damage. So can a hemorrhage inside the brain (**intracerebral hemorrhage**).

It is possible to suffer a major stroke either by a massive arterial occlusion or by an occlusion of a very small artery situated in a critical area. For instance, a sudden occlusion of the internal carotid artery may cause a massive cerebral infarction. An occlusion of one of the tiny arteries that arise from Willis' head (**medial striate, lateral striate**, or **anterior choroidal arteries** [a **lacunar infarct**]—**Figs. 2-2, 2-4**) may cause as much deficit by infarcting the **internal capsule**. The internal capsule is the narrow zone of a funnel of motor and sensory fibers that converge upon the brain stem from the cerebral cortex (**Fig. 2-8**). Each cerebral hemisphere contains one internal capsule, situated deep within the brain just behind Willis' head. The anterior choroidal artery and striate arteries supply the internal capsule and may hemorrhage in situations of hypertension or arteriosclerosis, thereby causing much damage from a tiny lesion.

The **ophthalmic artery** comes off the internal carotid artery near the posterior communicating artery. An occlusion of the internal carotid artery below this point can cause not only a hemispheric infarct on that side (with *contralateral* [opposite side of the body] weakness or sensory loss) but also blindness in the *ipsilateral* (same side) eye, which the ophthalmic artery supplies.

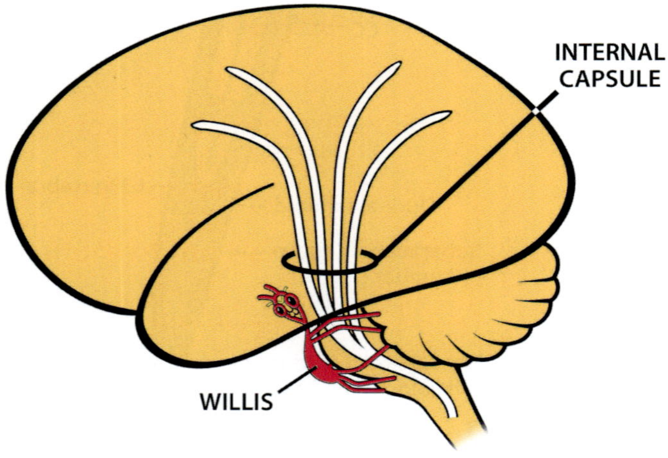


***Figure 2-8*** *Willis and the internal capsule.*

# 3

# Spinal Cord

The spinal cord, as seen in cross section (**Fig. 3-1**), contains central gray matter and peripheral white matter. The gray matter contains many neuronal cell bodies and synapses. The white matter contains ascending and descending axon pathways. The ascending pathways relay sensory information to the brain. The descending pathways relay motor instructions down from the brain. The number of synapses within a pathway is not very important to know clinically. However, it is vital to remember the sites of contralateral crossing over of the various pathways and the location of the pathways within the white matter as seen in cross section (**Figs. 3-1** and **3-2**).

## The Sites of Crossing Over

There are 3 main sensory systems entering the spinal cord:

1. Pain-temperature
2. Proprioception–stereognosis. *Proprioception* is the ability to sense the position of a body part without relying on vision. *Stereognosis* is the ability to recognize the form of an object by touch.
3. Light touch

To avoid confusion, no sensory synapses will be drawn in **Figure 3-2**. As a rule, though, there is a tendency for sensory fibers to synapse just prior to crossing over. For instance, the posterior columns, just prior to crossing over at the junction between spinal cord and brain stem, synapse in two nuclei: nucleus gracilis (from lower extremity) and nucleus cuneatus (from upper extremity).

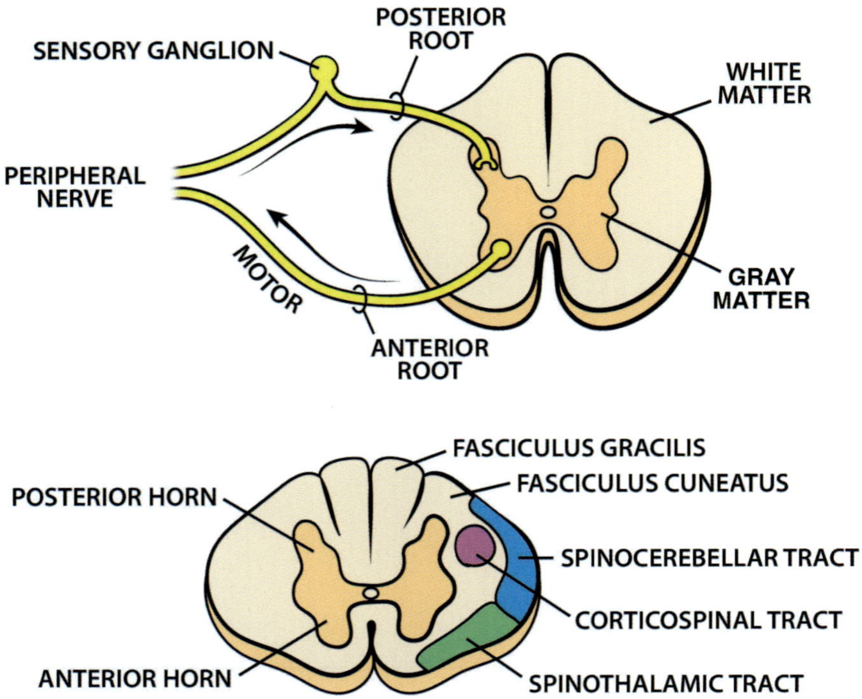


***Figure 3-1*** *Major subdivisions of the spinal cord. The posterior columns consist of the fasciculus gracilis plus fasciculus cuneatus.*

The pathway for pain and temperature enters the spinal cord, crosses over to the opposite half of the cord almost immediately (actually one or two spinal cord vertebral segments higher), ascends to the thalamus on the opposite side, and then moves on to the cerebral cortex. In reality, many fibers end in the brain stem and never make it as far as the thalamus, but these will not concern us here. A lesion of the spinothalamic tract will result in loss of pain-temperature sensation contralaterally, below the level of the lesion.

The pathway for proprioception and stereognosis (also for the perception of vibration), termed the posterior columns, initially remains on the same side of the spinal cord that it enters, crossing over at the junction between the spinal cord and brain stem. A lesion of the posterior columns in the spinal cord results in a decrease in conscious proprioception, stereognosis, and vibration ipsilaterally (same side) below the level of the lesion.

The path for light touch combines features of the above two pathways. It partly remains uncrossed until it reaches the level of the brain stem, and partly crosses over at lower levels. This is why light touch typically is spared in unilateral spinal cord lesions; there are alternate routes to carry the information.

All the above sensory pathways eventually cross over and terminate in the thalamus. From there, they are relayed to the sensory area of the cerebrum. A lesion of the sensory area of the cerebral cortex may result in a contralateral deficit of all the above sensory modalities.

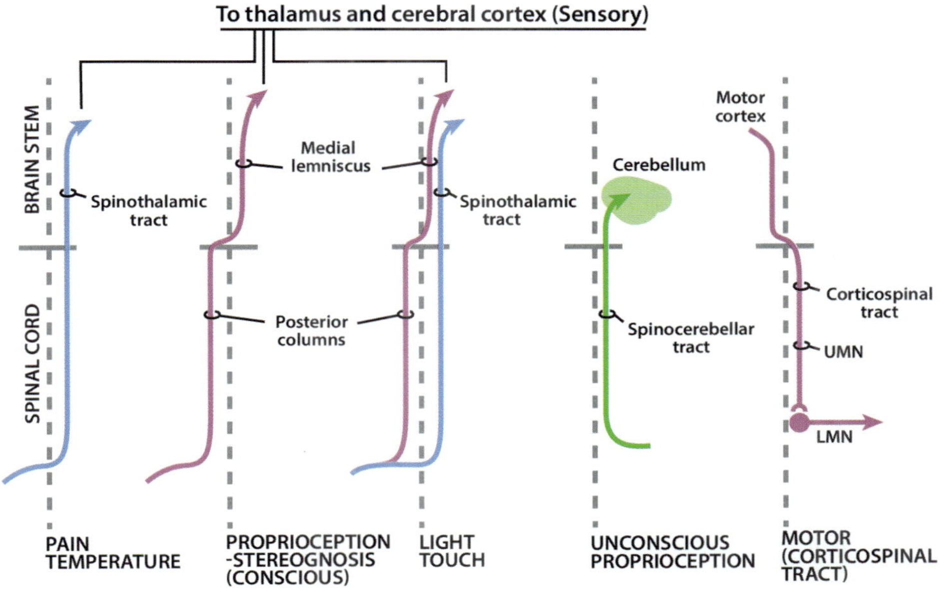


***Figure 3-2*** *Schematic view of the major ascending and descending pathways. UMN, upper motor neuron; LMN, lower motor neuron.*

Proprioception-stereognosis has a conscious and an unconscious component. The conscious pathway, mentioned above, connects with the thalamus and cerebral cortex, enabling you to describe, for instance, the position of your limb. The unconscious pathway connects with the cerebellum (the cerebellum is considered an unconscious organ) as the spinocerebellar pathway and enables you to walk and perform other complex acts subconsciously without having to think which joints are flexed and extended (**Fig. 3-3**). (In this book where it is stated that a patient presents with "proprioceptive loss," this refers to loss of conscious proprioceptive sensation, as tested by asking the patient to describe the position of a limb.)

Unlike the other sensory pathways, which cross contralaterally, the spinocerebellar primarily remains ipsilateral. In general, one side of the cerebellum connects with the same side of the body. Thus, *cerebellar lesions tend to produce ipsilateral malfunctioning, whereas cerebral lesions result in contralateral defects.*

The motor (corticospinal; pyramidal) pathway is relatively simple. It extends from the motor area of the cerebral cortex down through the brain stem, crossing over (i.e., decussates) at the pyramidal decussation at approximately the same level as the medial lemniscus (at the junction between brain stem and spinal cord) (**Figs. 3-2, 3-3**).

The corticospinal pathway synapses in the anterior horn (motor gray matter) of the spinal cord just prior to leaving the cord. This is that one synapse mentioned previously that is important to know about, for motor neurons above the level of this synapse (connecting the cerebral cortex and anterior horn) are termed upper motor neurons (UMN), whereas those beyond this level (the peripheral nerve neurons) are termed lower motor neurons

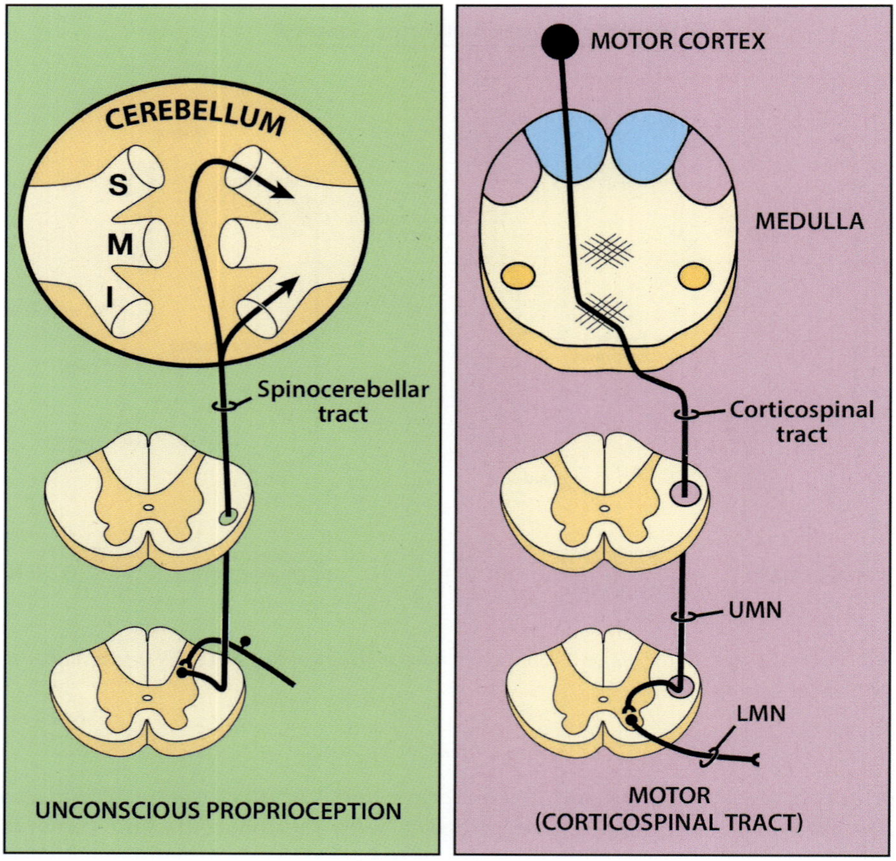


*Figure 3-3* *The spinocerebellar and corticospinal tracts. S., superior cerebellar peduncle; M., middle cerebellar peduncle; I., inferior cerebellar peduncle. UMN, upper motor neuron; LMN, lower motor neuron.*

(LMN). Upper and lower motor neuron injuries result in different clinical signs. Although both result in weakness, they differ as in **Figure 3-4**.

The caveat to the rules in **Figure 3-4**, is that right after injury, everything might look floppy - wait and see what develops.

| FIGURE 3-4 UPPER AND LOWER MOTOR NEURON WEAKNESS | |
|---|---|
| **Upper Motor Neuron Defect (Brain/Spinal Cord Problem)** | **Lower Motor Neuron Defect (Nerve/Muscle Problem)** |
| • Weak BUT reflexes work (may be incr.) | • Weak AND reflexes don't work |
| • Muscles don't shrink much | • Muscles shrink (atrophy) |
| • No muscle twitching (fasciculations) | • Muscles twitch |
| • Babinski sign (big toe goes up) | • No Babinski sign |
| • Think: Stroke, spinal cord injury, multiple sclerosis | • Think: Pinched nerve, nerve damage |

## Cross-Sectional Location of the Pathways

**Figure 3-1** illustrates the positions of the sensory and motor pathways in cross section.

For largely unclear reasons, various diseases affect different portions of the spinal cord. **Amyotrophic lateral sclerosis (ALS, Lou Gehrig's disease) (Fig. 3-5A)** is characterized by a combination of upper and lower motor neuron signs—muscle weakness, atrophy, fibrillations, and fasciculations combined with hyperreflexia. The lesion involves both the anterior horns (motor) of the gray matter (a lower motor neuron lesion) as well as the corticospinal tracts (an upper motor neuron lesion).

**Tertiary syphilis** (tabes dorsalis) includes proprioceptive loss and pain (posterior root irritation), particularly affecting the lower extremities. The lesion involves the posterior columns of white matter (**Fig. 3-5B**) and may extend to the posterior roots and root ganglia.

In **pernicious anemia (Fig. 3-5C)**, there is proprioceptive loss and upper motor neuron weakness. The lesion involves the posterior columns and corticospinal tracts.

**Polio** attacks the anterior horn cells (**Fig. 3-5D**), leading to lower motor neuron involvement, with weakness, atrophy, fasciculations, fibrillations, and hyporeflexia.

Individuals with **Guillain-Barré syndrome** (**Fig. 3-5E**) experience sensory and lower motor neuron loss because of peripheral nerve involvement.

In **syringomyelia (Fig. 3-5F)**, there is a defect at the center of the cord that interrupts the crossing of the pain-temperature fibers of the spinothalamic tract. If the lesion is large enough, it may also affect nearby areas in the spinal cord. The patient may have, for instance, bilateral paralysis below the level of the lesion from interruption of the nearby corticospinal tracts, fasciculations and muscle atrophy at the level of C8T1 from interruption of the anterior gray matter at that level, as well as decreased pain-temperature sensation at that level from interruption of the crossing pain-temperature fibers.

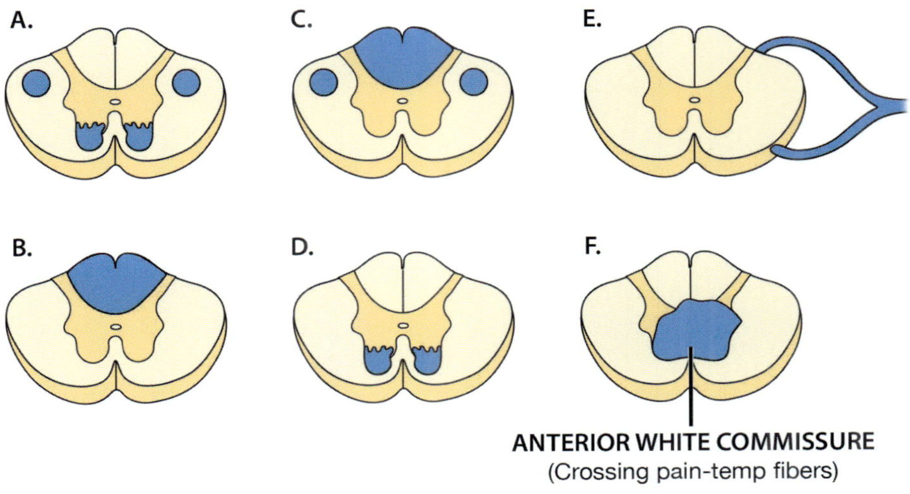


***Figure 3-5*** *Lesions sites in classical diseases. A. Amyotrophic lateral sclerosis (Lou Gehrig's disease). B. Tertiary syphilis. C. Pernicious anemia. D. Polio. E. Guillain-Barré. F. Syringomyelia.*

The **anterior spinal artery**, which arises from Willis (**Fig. 2-5**) supplies the anterior part of the spinal cord, leaving the posterior columns unaffected. The **posterior spinal arteries**, which arise near the anterior spinal artery, supply the posterior columns. Thus, an anterior spinal artery occlusion may affect all the spinal pathways except for the posterior columns. A posterior spinal artery occlusion has its main detrimental effects on the posterior columns.

Certain muscle groups may be affected more than others in an upper motor neuron lesion. In the typical cerebral hemisphere stroke secondary to carotid artery occlusion, the patient develops **decorticate posturing**, characterized by flexion of the wrist and elbow and extension (straightening) of the ankle and knee. In midbrain strokes, the posturing is similar, except that the elbow is extended (**decerebrate posturing**). The mechanisms apparently involve injury to other motor pathways (extrapyramidal) outside the corticospinal (pyramidal) system. "Pure" lesions of the corticospinal tract result predominantly in difficulty with skilled movements of the distal aspect of the extremities.

The pathways mentioned above belong to the somatic motor and somatic sensory systems. Somatic motor fibers innervate striated skeletal muscle. Somatic sensory fibers innervate predominantly the skin, muscle, and tissues other than the viscera. "**Viscera**" means cardiac muscle, smooth muscle (as in the gut) and glands. Visceral (autonomic) motor cells are located in the gray matter between the somatic sensory and motor areas of the spinal cord gray matter (**Fig. 3-1**).

# 4

# Brain Stem

The main functions of the 12 cranial nerves:

CN1: (Olfactory nerve) Smells
CN2: (Optic nerve) Sees
**CN3**: (Oculomotor nerve) Moves eye medially (medial rectus muscle); constricts pupils; accommodates
**CN4**: (Trochlear nerve) Moves eye down and out (superior oblique muscle)
**CN6**: (Abducens nerve) Moves eye laterally (lateral rectus muscle)
CN5: (Trigeminal nerve) Chews (masseter muscle) and feels front of head (like a face mask)
CN7: (Facial nerve) Moves the face, tastes (anterior 2/3 of the tongue), cries (lacrimates), and spits (salivates)
CN8: (Vestibulocochlear nerve) Hears, regulates balance
CN9: (Glossopharyngeal nerve) Tastes (posterior 1/3 of the tongue), salivates, swallows, monitors carotid body and sinus
CN10: (Vagus nerve) Swallows, lifts palate, talks (controls the larynx), communication to and from thoraco-abdominal viscera, down to the splenic flexure of the large colon
CN11: (Accessory nerve) Turns head, lifts shoulders
CN12: (Glossopharyngeal nerve) Moves tongue (to the opposite side of the nerve)

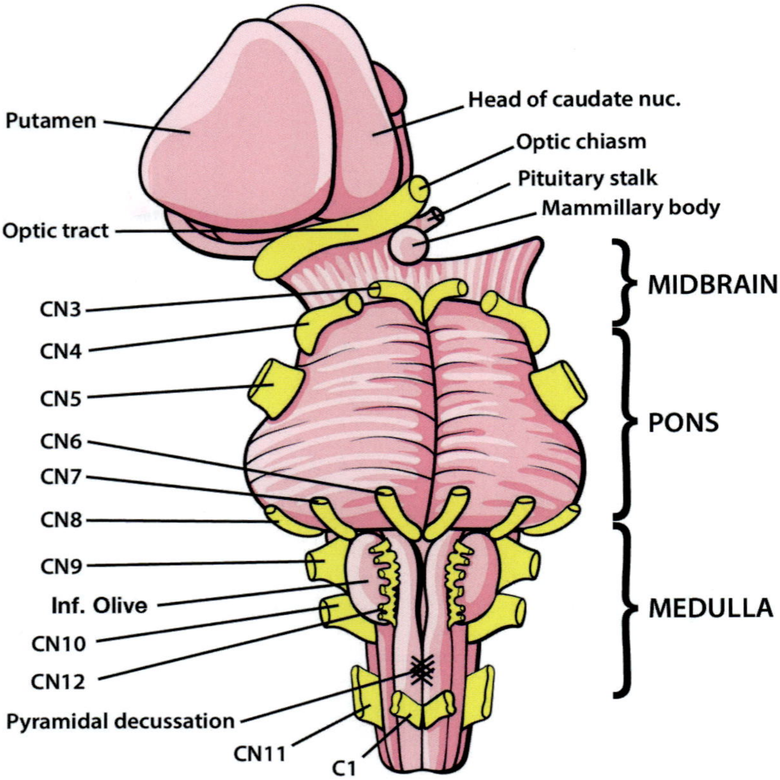


*Figure 4-1* The base (ventral view) of the brain stem.

The 12 cranial nerves and their nuclei are apportioned fairly equally between the 3 brain stem segments (CNs 1, 2, 3, 4 in midbrain; CNs 5, 6, 7, 8 in pons; CNs 9, 10, 11, 12 in medulla). Actually, that's not quite true. CNs 1 and 2 lie not in the midbrain but more rostrally near the diencephalon (**Fig. 4-2**). Also, although all divisions of CN5 enter the pons, the sensory nucleus of CN5 extends from midbrain to upper spinal cord (**Fig. 4-3**); the nuclei of CN8 lie not only in the pons but also in the medulla; the nuclei and nerve entry points of CN7 are located in both pons and medulla. These exceptions for CNs 5, 7, and 8 are indicated in parentheses in **Figure 4-2**. Lesions in the brain stem may damage the cranial nerves or their nuclei in these approximate locations.

In general, the cranial nerves exit near the base (ventral surface) of the brain stem; their nuclei and projecting nerves all are located and exit on the same side of the brain stem, without crossing over. The only clinically important exception to this is dumb CN4 (trochlear nerve), which both crosses over and passes over the roof of the brain stem. No wonder CN4 was delegated the most insignificant of all the cranial nerve functions, that of moving the superior oblique muscle.

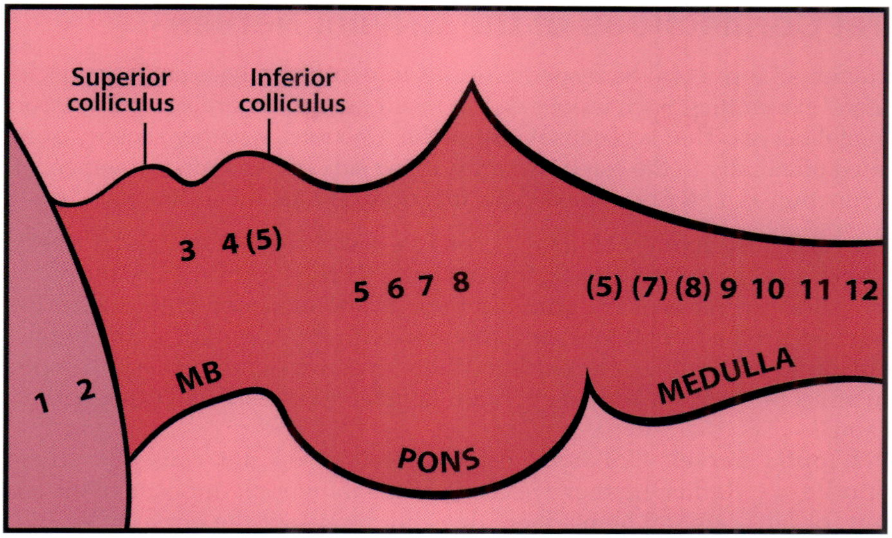


*Figure 4-2* The location of the cranial nerves and their nuclei within the midbrain (MB), pons, and medulla as seen laterally.

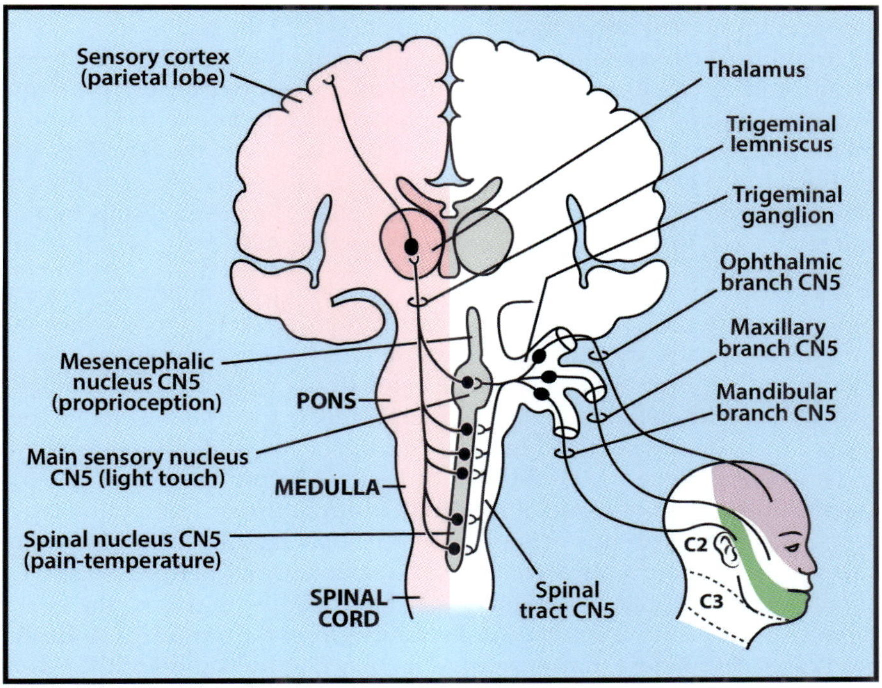


*Figure 4-3* Central sensory connections of the trigeminal nerve. The spinal nucleus of CN5 extends from the pons to spinal level C2.

## Central Connections of the Cranial Nerves

Destruction of a cerebral hemisphere results in dense paralysis and sensory loss in the contralateral extremities. Such lesions do not result in contralateral loss of function of most of the cranial nerves. That is because most of the functions, whether sensory or motor, are represented bilaterally in the cerebral cortex; if one side of the brain is damaged, the other side can function as a backup. The deficits that do result are the following:

- **CN1 (olfactory nerve)**: Unilateral cerebral lesions cause unilateral anosmia (loss of smell), because CN1 does not cross over. It runs from the nasal cavity through the cribriform plate of the ethmoid bone to the olfactory bulb, which lies on the underside of the frontal lobe, and connects with the same side of the brain. Since its pathway runs near the optic chiasm (Willis' eyebrows), tumors near the optic chiasm can affect both vision and smell. Brain damage near CN1 will cause ipsilateral loss of smell.
- **CN2 (optic nerve)**: Unilateral cerebral lesions do not cause blindness in the opposite eye. Rather, neither eye can see the *environment* opposite to the lesion. The right (or left) cerebral hemisphere does not represent the opposite eye, but rather the opposite environment (opposite visual field), which each eye can normally see (**Fig. 5-1**).
- **CNs 3, 4, and 6** (nerves to the eye muscles): Unilateral cerebral lesions do not cause paralysis of the opposite individual eye muscles, but paralysis of horizontal gaze of both eyes toward the opposite environment. It seems that the brain represents the opposite environment rather than the opposite side of the body.
- **CN5 (trigeminal nerve)**: Sensory fibers of CN5 enter the brain stem at the level of the pons and end up crossing over to eventually reach the opposite cerebral hemisphere, A lesion destroying one cerebral hemisphere will interfere with sensation coming from the opposite side of the body and the opposite side of the face (**Fig. 4-3**).
- **CN7 (facial nerve)**: Damage to the facial nerve causes paralysis of the entire face on the same side. Damage to a cerebral hemisphere, however, results in only partial paralysis of CN7, that of the opposite *lower* face (**Fig. 4-4**).

**Figure 4-4** illustrates the clinical difference between upper motor neuron and lower motor neuron damage to CN7. If a lesion severs CN7 (lesion seen in red), which innervates the upper and lower face, that entire side of the face becomes paralyzed. The forehead on the affected side appears ironed out. The eye will not close and there is flattening of the nasolabial fold with inability to smile on that side. If the lesion is above the level of the nucleus of CN7 (lesion seen in blue), i.e., an upper motor neuronal lesion, e.g., in a stroke of the cerebral cortex, only the area of the face below the eyes (on the opposite side) is paralyzed because of bilateral innervation of the upper face by the two cerebral hemispheres. A patient with this cerebral lesion has no significant difficulty closing the eyes. However, the patient with **Bell's palsy**, a spontaneous peripheral nerve 7 palsy, commonly of unknown etiology (perhaps viral), has difficulty in closing the eyes, because CN7 innervates the orbicularis oculus muscle, which closes the eyes (**Figs. 4-4B** and **4-5**). In pronounced cases, the patient may even need a tarsorrhaphy (suture of the lids together) to prevent drying out of the eye. Fortunately, Bell's palsy usually improves within a few weeks or months on corticosteroids (to reduce inflammation of the facial nerve), lubricating eye drops, and an eye patch.

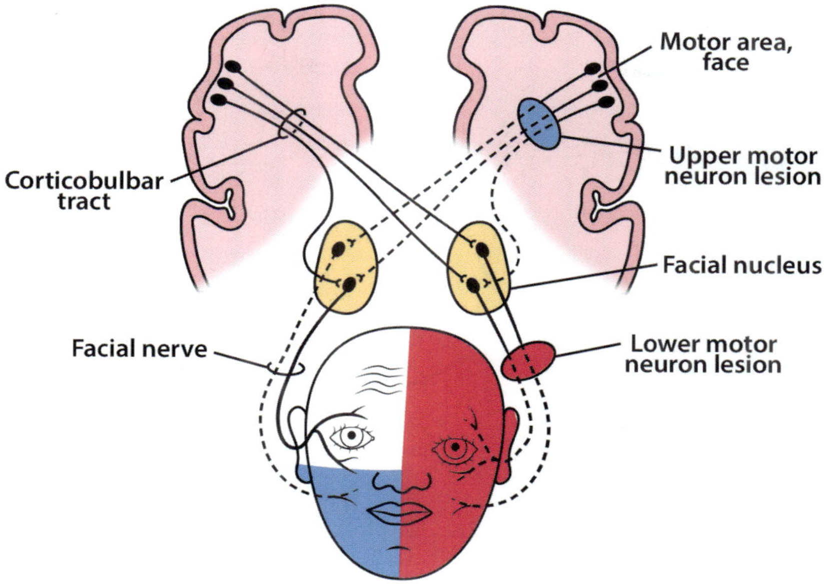


*Figure 4-4* *Facial paralysis caused by upper and lower motor lesions of the facial nerve (CN7). Shaded facial areas indicate zones of facial paralysis.*

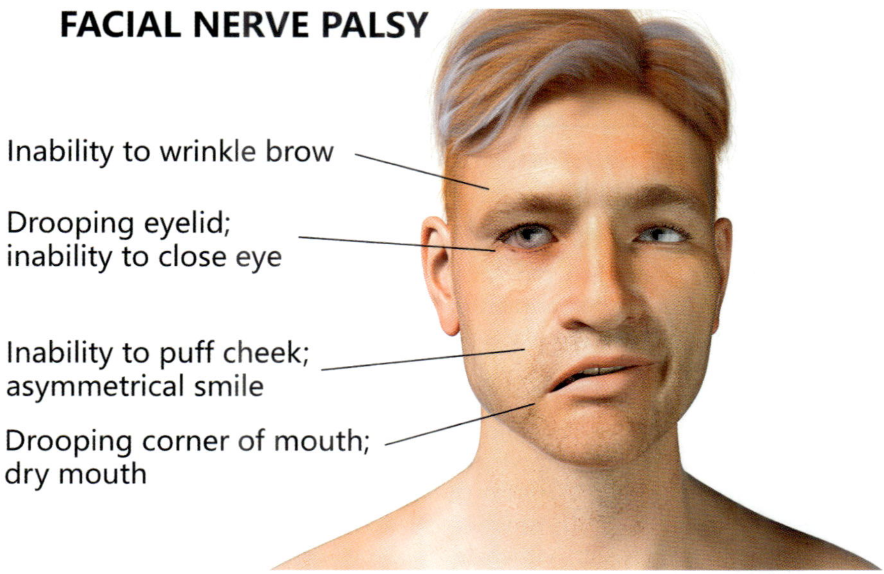


*Figure 4-4B* *Facial paralysis in Bell's palsy.*

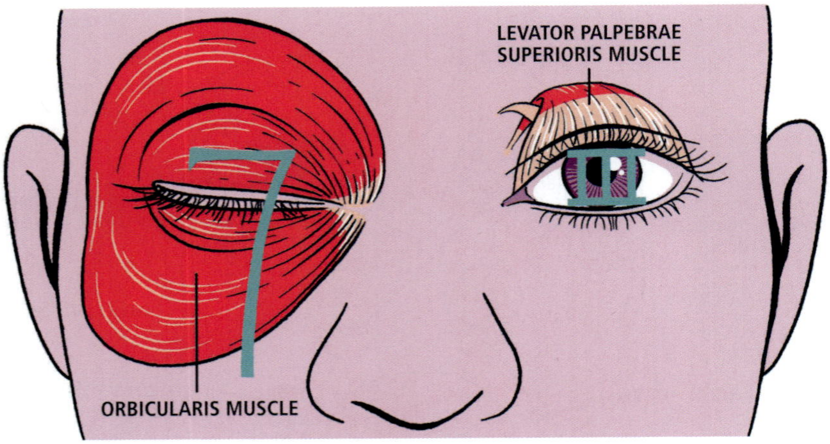


*Figure 4-5* *Eyelid innervations of CNs 7 and 3. The facial nerve (CN7), a "hook," closes the eye. The oculomotor nerve (CN3), "three pillars" opens the eyes.*

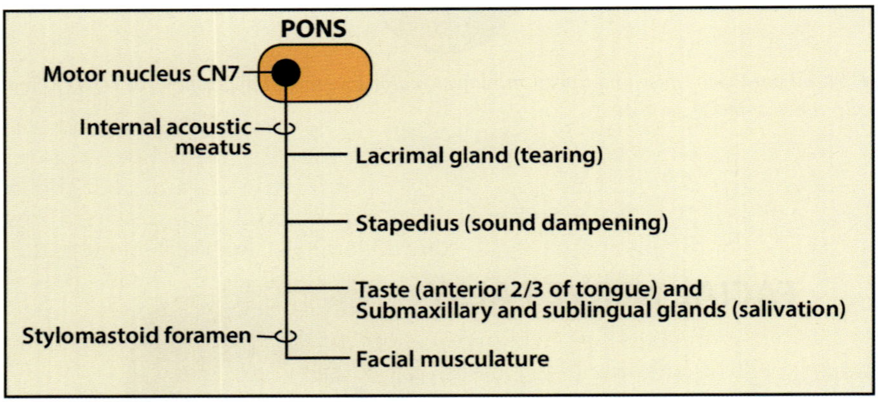


*Figure 4-6* *Schematic view of the course of CN7.*

**Ramsay-Hunt syndrome** is a type of Bell's palsy caused by varicella-zoster virus, the same virus found in chickenpox and shingles. In addition to facial nerve paralysis, it may present with pain and shingles blisters around the external ear or farther along the facial nerve distribution.

The usual site of injury in Bell's palsy is somewhere in the facial canal (which lies between the *internal acoustic meatus* and the *stylomastoid foramen* (**Fig. 4-6**) and may involve other branches of CN7 (to the stapedius muscle, lacrimal and salivary glands). Since the stapedius dampens sound waves, its nonfunctioning leads to hyperacusis, wherein sounds appear excessively loud. Usually, function returns after Bell's palsy. The patient may then experience "crocodile tears," in which the patient tears on eating, instead of salivating, owing to misguided growth of the regenerating salivary and lacrimal fibers.

- **CN8 (vestibulocochlear nerve):** Unilateral cerebral lesions do not cause deafness (CN8) or significant loss of CN 9, 10, or 11 function because these nerves are represented bilaterally in the brain. If one side of the brain is injured, the opposite hemisphere acts as a backup to maintain function. Thus, deafness in one ear likely results from either a lesion to the nerve or to the peripheral auditory apparatus (e.g., eardrum or cochlear nucleus in the inner ear).
- **CN12 (hypoglossal nerve):** Unilateral cerebral lesion may cause weakness of the opposite side of the tongue.

Thus, the main cranial nerve functions that may be lost in a cerebral lesion are loss of sensation in the opposite face, weakness of the opposite lower face, weakness of the opposite tongue, and loss of ability to see the opposite environment or move the eyes toward the opposite environment. If other cranial nerve functions are involved, suspect that the lesion lies in the periphery, either to the cranial nerve, its nucleus in the brain stem, or its receptor (e.g., the outer or inner ear).

## The Long Tracts

The main pathways through the brain stem are illustrated in **Figure 4-7**. The **corticospinal tract**, medial lemniscus, spinothalamic tract, and spinocerebellar tracts are the most important clinically. Not shown is the **corticobulbar tract**, which accompanies the corticospinal tract and stops off to connect with the various brain stem motor nuclei. Unilateral damage to the corticobulbar tract does not cause massive cranial nerve dysfunction because each tract connects bilaterally with most cranial nerve motor nuclei. If one corticobulbar tract is damaged, the other tract carries on the function. The important exceptions are CNs 7 and 12, as corticobulbar tract lesions result in contralateral lower facial paralysis (**Fig. 4-4**) and, in some patients, contralateral weakness of the tongue. *Bilateral* lesions of the corticobulbar tracts result in a profound dysfunction, termed **pseudobulbar palsy**. Patients with this disorder have trouble not only with facial expression and motion of the tongue, but with chewing, swallowing, speech, and breathing. There may also be inappropriate spells of laughing or crying as part of the syndrome.

For practical clinical purposes, one may assume that corticobulbar fibers cross over to the opposite side of the brain stem at about the same brain stem level as their motor nuclei of termination.

The topographical arrangement of HAL (Head, Arm, Leg) is better known for the medial lemniscus than the other fiber pathways. Picture Mr. HAL standing upright in the medial lemniscus of the medulla (**Fig. 4-7**). On approaching the sleep area in higher brain centers he gets sleepier and sleepier until he is lying down at the level of the midbrain.

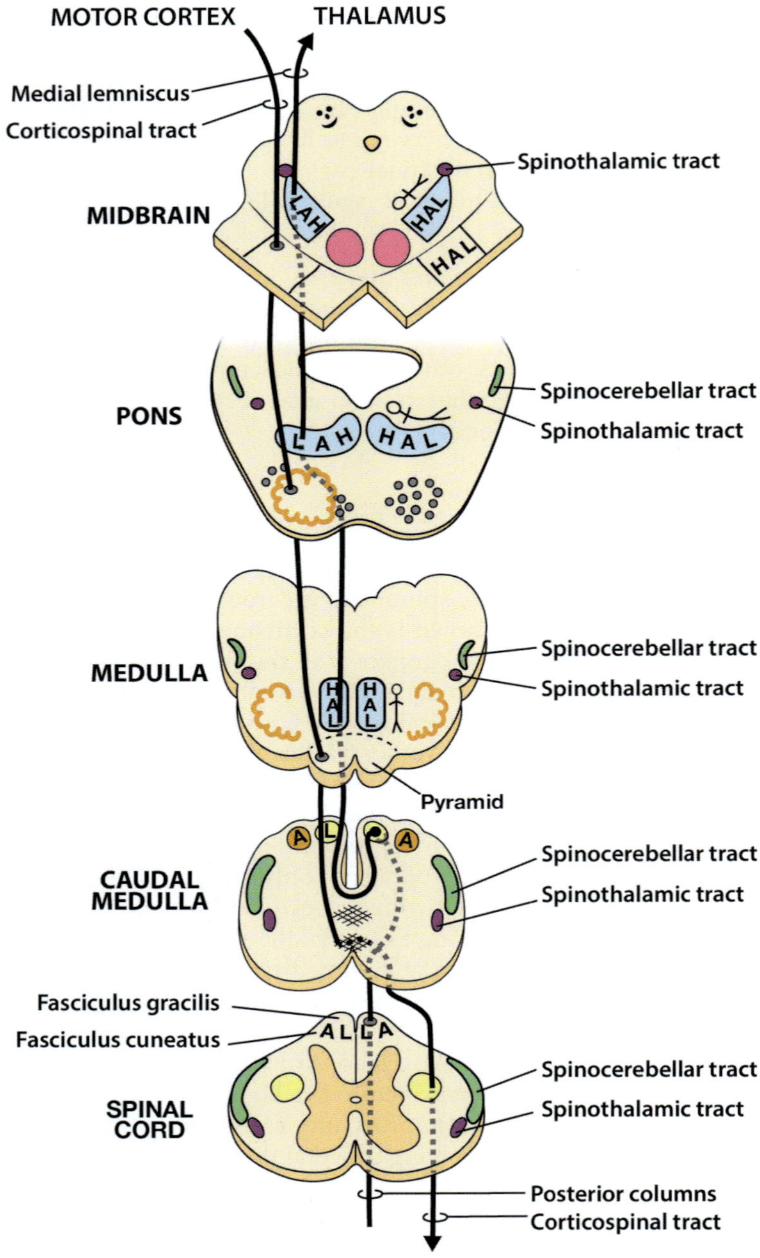


***Figure 4-7*** *The location of the major fiber pathways in the spinal cord and brain stem. HAL = Head, Arm, Leg.*

# 5

# Visual System

Optic fibers temporal to the fovea connect with the brain ipsilaterally (same side). Fibers nasal to the fovea cross over to the opposite side at the optic chiasm to connect contralaterally (opposite side). A lesion of the optic tract on the left, therefore, results in loss of the right visual field in each eye.

Note (**Fig. 5-1**) that the right visual field falls on the left half of each retina; the superior visual field falls on the inferior retina. The right visual field projects to the left side of the brain. The superior visual field projects below the calcarine fissure in the occipital lobe. In other words, everything is upside down and backwards, provided you think in terms of visual fields. For example, a patient with a lesion below the left calcarine fissure experiences a right superior field deficit (**Fig. 5-1**).

The center of the retina (the fovea, which is the area of most acute vision) projects to the tip of the occipital lobe (**Fig. 5-2**). Thus, a patient with a severe blow to the back of the head may experience bilateral central scotomas (visual field defects) if both occipital poles are destroyed.

Commonly, visual field defects partially spare the macula (the area of retina in the immediate vicinity of the fovea). This may be due to the large representation of the macula on the visual cortex, with overlapping blood supplies, resulting in only partial lesions. It may also be due to artifacts of eye fixation during the exam, or to a certain degree of bilateral representation of the macula.

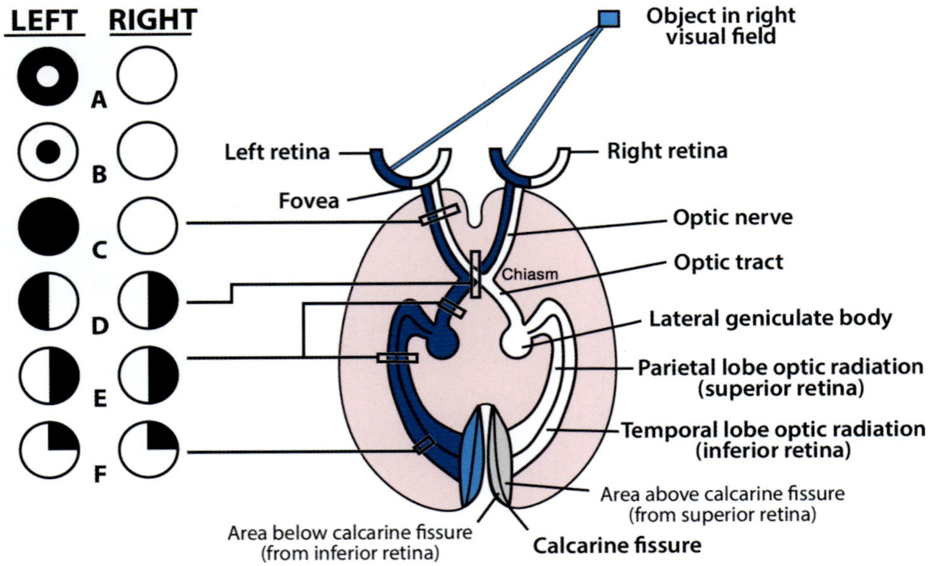


***Figure 5-1*** *The visual pathways as seen from above the brain. Letters A-F refer to visual field defects following lesions in the corresponding brain areas. Circles indicate what the left and right eyes see. Black areas represent visual field defects. A. Constricted field left eye (e.g., end-stage glaucoma). When constricted fields are bilateral, it may signify a nonphysiological condition. B. Central scotoma (e.g., optic neuritis in multiple sclerosis; macular degeneration), C. Total blindness of the left eye. D. Bitemporal hemianopia (e.g., pituitary gland tumor). E. Right homonymous hemianopia (e.g., stroke). F. Right superior quadrantanopia (from lesion below the calcarine fissure).*

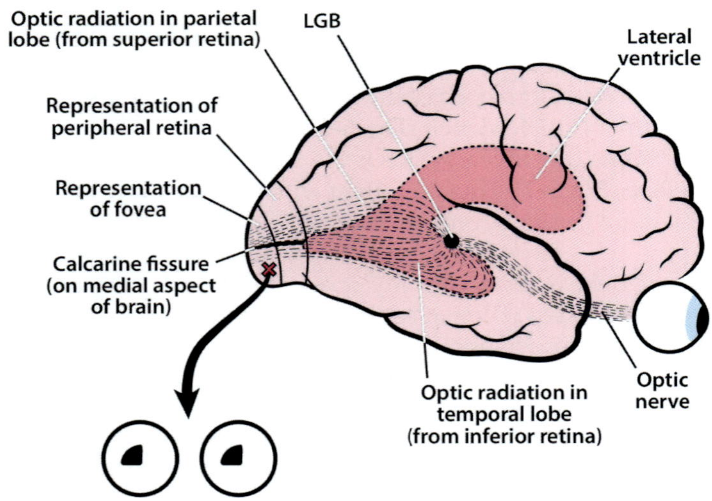


***Figure 5-2*** *Lateral view of the visual pathways, showing the visual field defect resulting from a lesion below the right calcarine fissure in the foveal region of the occipital cortex. LGB, lateral geniculate body.*

## Optic Reflexes: Pupillary Constriction to Light

Unlike the pathways mediating vision, which involve a synapse in the lateral geniculate body (a part of the thalamus), the pupillary light reflex involves a direct pathway to the rostral midbrain from the optic tract (**Fig. 5-3**). The rostral midbrain looks like a double-headed gingerbread man. Shining a light in one eye normally leads to constriction of both pupils (termed the *consensual reflex*) as may be deduced from the connections depicted in **Figure 5-3**.

## Accommodation

Accommodation (**Fig. 5-3**) involves a neural circuit to the visual cortex and back, which makes sense, for we need our cerebral cortex to determine that something is out of focus before we can send directions to correct the focus. Focusing occurs by stimulating the

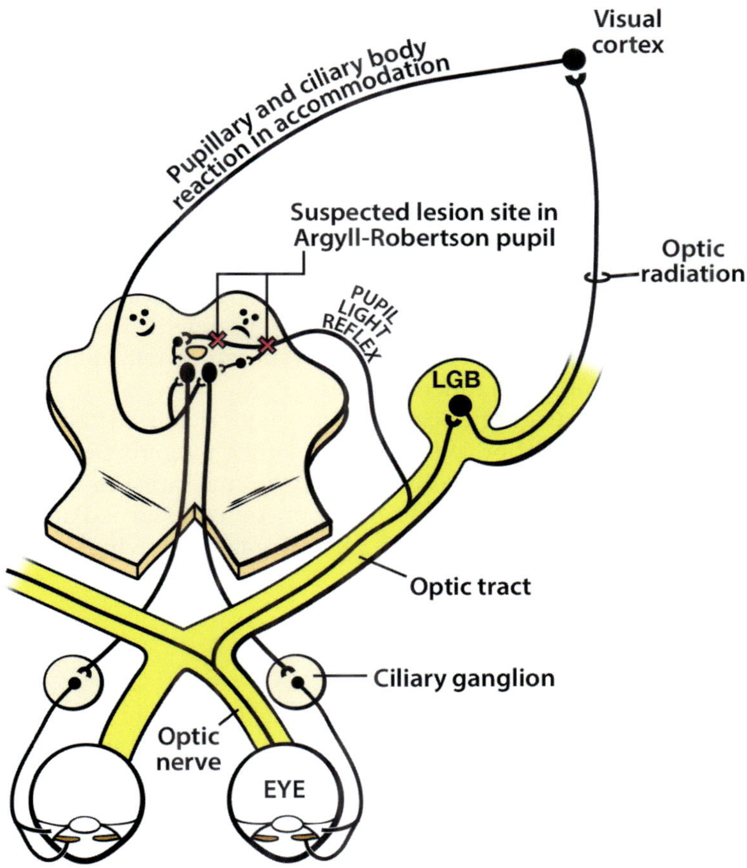


*Figure 5-3 The pathways for the pupillary light reflex and accommodation in the rostral midbrain. LGB, lateral geniculate body. The light reflex pathway involves only pupillary constriction, whereas the accommodation pathway affects both pupillary constriction and ciliary body accommodation.*

smooth muscle of the ciliary body in the eye to contract, thereby enabling the lens to change its shape (*accommodation*). During accommodation not only does the lens focus but the pupil constricts, both smooth muscle actions mediated by parasympathetic components of CN3.

The syphilitic (Argyll-Robertson) pupil (also called the prostitute's pupil because it accommodates but does not react) constricts during accommodation, which is normal, but does not constrict to light. The lesion is considered to lie in the pretectal area of the superior colliculus (face of the gingerbread man in **Fig. 5-3**).

## Conjugate Gaze

Damage to the motor areas of the cerebral cortex produces contralateral paralysis of the extremities. It does not produce loss of all the contralateral eye muscle movements, but rather loss of the ability of either eye to look toward the contralateral environment. Following a lesion to the left visuomotor area (Brodmann's area 8 in the frontal lobe —see **Fig. 8-1**), the patient cannot voluntarily look to the right. His eyes tend to deviate to the left. They are said to "look at the lesion." This occurs because the pathway from the left hemisphere innervates the right lateral rectus muscle (right CN6) and the left medial rectus muscle (left CN3)(**Fig. 5-4**). The right lateral rectus and left medial rectus muscles both direct the eyes to the right.

A lesion to the medial longitudinal fasciculus bilaterally, most commonly seen in multiple sclerosis, would produce a decreased ability for either eye to look medially (**Figs. 5-4** and **5-5**). In this instance, both eyes can converge because the pathway for convergence (as well as vertical gaze) is different from the path for lateral conjugate gaze. The condition resulting from lesions to the MLF is known as the MLF (medial longitudinal fasciculus) syndrome, or **internuclear ophthalmoplegia** (**Fig. 5-5**).

In the **one-and-a-half syndrome**, there is a lesion of one abducens (CN6) nucleus, as well as the crossed connections to both MLFs. Thus, in a right-sided lesion, neither eye can look to the right on attempted right conjugate gaze. On attempted left conjugate gaze, only the left eye moves, as its lateral rectus function is preserved.

Convergence and vertical gaze apparently involve circuits in the midbrain close to (although not within) the superior colliculus (face of the gingerbread man in **Figure 5-3**). Hence, difficulty with convergence and vertical gaze may arise in tumors of the pineal gland that press upon the brain stem at the superior collicular level. **Parinaud's syndrome** is pupillary constriction and paralysis of vertical gaze following lesions close to the superior colliculus.

## Nystagmus

Nystagmus is a repetitive, tremor-like oscillating movement of the eyes. The most common form of nystagmus is **horizontal jerk nystagmus**, where the eyes repetitively move slowly toward one side and then quickly back. It is normal to have a slight degree of such nystagmus on attempted extreme lateral gaze, but marked degrees are abnormal and found in a variety of clinical conditions. **Vertical nystagmus** is always abnormal, signifying a disorder in brain stem function. **Pendular nystagmus**, in which the eye moves at equal speeds in both directions, commonly is congenital or present after prolonged periods of blindness.

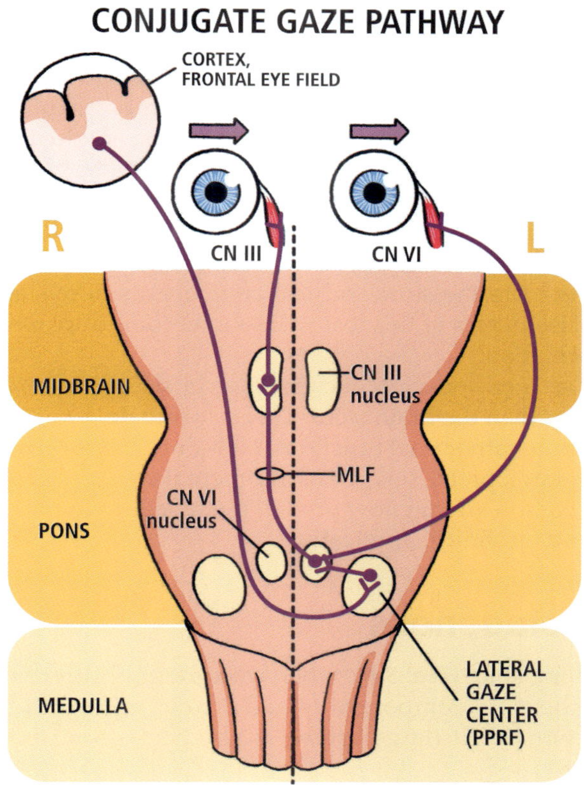


***Figure 5-4*** *The pathway for lateral conjugate gaze, originating from areas 8, 17, 18, and 19 of the cerebral cortex (see* **Fig. 8-1***). PPRF—pontine paramedian reticular formation. Nuc. 3, nucleus of CN3. Nuc. 6, nucleus of CN6.*

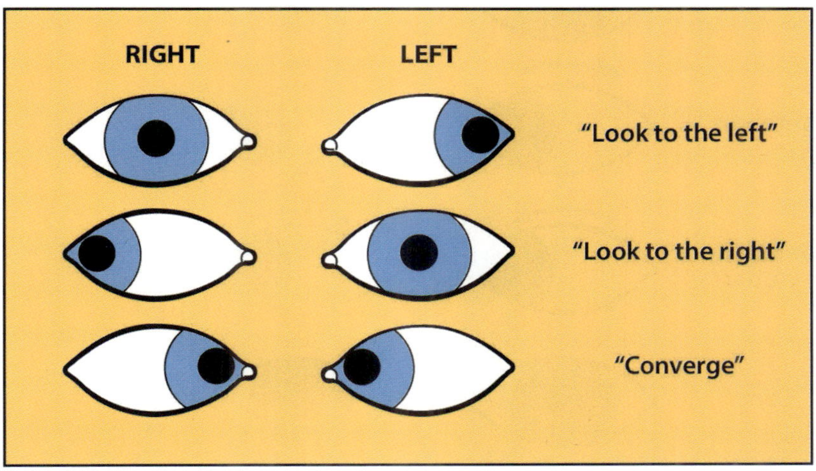


***Figure 5-5*** *MLF syndrome. Medial rectus does not contract during lateral gaze but does contract on convergence.*

The pathways for nystagmus are so complicated that the situation is best explained by a little story.

It is common knowledge that the brain stem is very dumb and slow, being the most primitive part of the brain. The cerebral cortex, a relatively recent evolutionary development, is smart and fast. One day, a man was driving along in his car when someone sitting to his right squirted some cold water into his right ear (the clinical test known as **cold calorics**). The dumb brain stem sluggishly moved its eyes to the right, drawling in its deep, slow tone "HEY-Y-Y-Y-Y! WHO'S SQUIRTING COLD WATER IN MY EAR?" Alarmed at this, the smart, quick cortex quickly jerked the eyes back, shouting "HEY! GET BACK AND LOOK AT THE ROAD!" These are the slow and fast components of nystagmus following cold calorics. The clinical usefulness of this test will soon become apparent, after the following bit of additional information.

We all know that as consciousness declines, say in sleep, the cerebral cortex becomes depressed more readily than the brain stem. This is fortunate, for if the brain stem went to sleep we might lose some rather vital functions, like control of respiration, which is located in the brain stem. It takes a pretty severe environmental change to depress the brain stem. With the above information we can now predict the reflex ocular responses to cold caloric testing and understand its clinical application.

## State of Consciousness

In the normal waking state (**Fig. 5-6**), when cold water is introduced into the ear there is nystagmus, with the slow component (small arrow) toward the side of stimulation, followed by a fast component (large arrow) in the opposite direction. There is no net

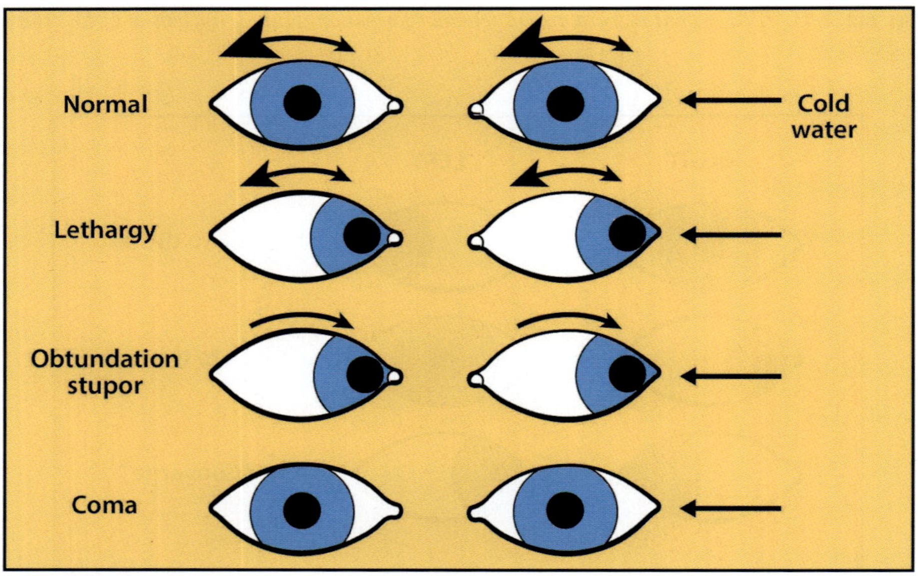


***Figure 5-6*** *Cold caloric responses in states of altered consciousness. Small arrow indicates the slow phase of nystagmus. Large arrow indicates the fast phase.*

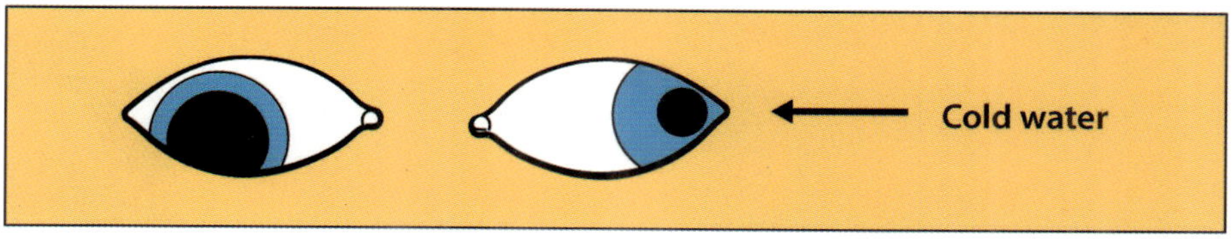


*Figure 5-7* Cold calorics in a case of right CN3 paralysis.

deviation of the eyes. As the patient becomes lethargic, the cortex begins to fall asleep first, so the fast component of nystagmus becomes less pronounced. There still is nystagmus but also a net deviation of the eyes toward the cold water. With further depression (obtundation, stupor) there is deviation without the fast movement of nystagmus, for the cerebral component is defective. With coma, the brain stem becomes depressed and there is no movement at all. Whereas the last pattern occurs in true coma, the first pattern appears in a patient faking coma.

## Muscle Paresis

Cold calorics can confirm the suspicion of a CN3 or CN6 paresis in a stuporous patient (**Fig. 5-7**). For instance, the uncus, a portion of the temporal lobe lying particularly close to CN3 (**Fig. 2-4**) may herniate against CN3 and damage it after a subdural hemorrhage, resulting in a widely dilated, fixed (unresponsive to light) pupil. (The pupil also points down and out due to unrestricted contraction of the superior oblique muscle.) Cold calorics, by confirming the presence of medial rectus weakness, helps to confirm that the dilated pupil is due to CN3 injury and not to other causes (e.g., someone placing dilating drops in the eye and not telling anyone).

## Doll's Eye Phenomenon

On turning the head suddenly to one side there is a tendency in patients without brain stem damage for the eyes to lag behind. This is the **Doll's Eye phenomenon**, as in a doll's eye which looks down when the head is tilted back. The reflex is believed to be brain stem mediated and any asymmetry or lack of response is believed to reflect significant brain stem dysfunction. Of course, it is wise to know, before performing this exam, that the patient does not have a broken neck.

# 6

# Autonomic System and Hypothalamus

The autonomic system regulates glands, smooth muscle and cardiac muscle. It contains sympathetic and parasympathetic components. The sympathetic system as a whole is a **catabolic system**, expending energy, as in the flight-or-fight response to danger, e.g., increasing the heart rate and contractility and shunting blood to the muscles and heart. The parasympathetic system is an **anabolic system**, conserving energy, e.g., in slowing the heart rate and in promoting the digestion and absorption of food. The cell bodies of preganglionic sympathetic fibers lie in the intermediolateral columns of the spinal cord at spinal cord levels T1-L2 (**Figs. 6-1A, 6-2**). Those of the parasympathetic system occupy comparable positions at spinal cord levels S2-S4 (**Figs. 6-1B, 6-2**).

In addition, cranial nerves 3, 7, 9 and 10 have parasympathetic components (CN3—pupil and ciliary body constriction; CN 7—tearing and salivation; CN9—salivation; CN10—the vagus and its ramifications).

In order to extend all over the body, the sympathetic system fibers leave the spinal cord at levels T1-L2, enter the paravertebral ganglion chain and then may travel up or down the chain for considerable distances prior to synapsing (**Fig. 6-2**). The sympathetic chain stretches from the foramen magnum to the coccyx and supplies the far reaches of the body with post-ganglionic sympathetic fibers. Parasympathetic fibers reach widespread areas via CN10, the vagus nerve (**Fig. 6-2**).

Both parasympathetic and sympathetic systems contain two neurons between the spinal cord and periphery. The first synapse in the parasympathetic or sympathetic system is cholinergic (containing acetylcholine). For the sympathetic system this synapse is either

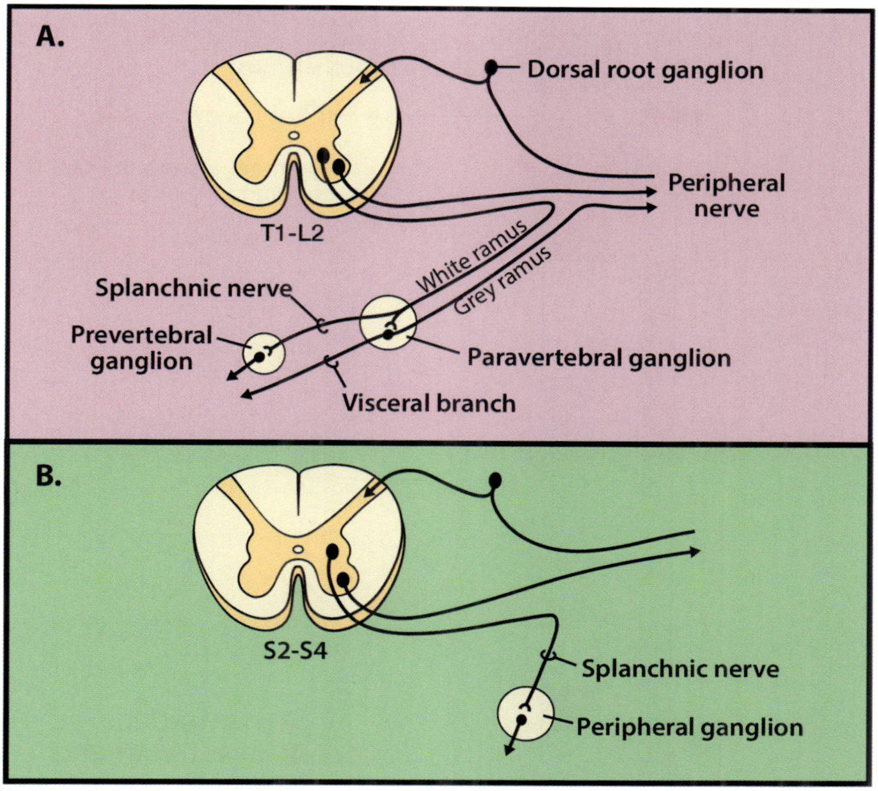


***Figure 6-1*** *A. The sympathetic nerve routes. B. The parasympathetic nerve routes.*

in the paravertebral chain of sympathetic ganglia or farther away in the prevertebral ganglion plexuses (**Fig. 6-1A**).

Parasympathetic synapses typically lie very close to or within the viscera. The final synapse of the parasympathetic system contains acetylcholine. The final synapse of the sympathetic system contains noradrenaline, except for certain synapses, as for sweating, that contain acetylcholine (i.e., are cholinergic). In **Figure 6-3**, note that secretory functions in general are stimulated by cholinergic fibers.

In extreme fear both systems may act simultaneously, producing involuntary emptying of the bladder and rectum (parasympathetic) along with a generalized sympathetic response. In more pleasant circumstances, namely in sexual arousal, the parasympathetic system mediates penile and clitoral erection and the sympathetic controls ejaculation.

Proceeding rostrally from the caudal tip of the spinal cord, one first finds a parasympathetic area (S2-S4), followed by a sympathetic region (T1-L2), then parasympathetic areas (CNs 10, 9, 7, 3) and then, successively, a sympathetic and parasympathetic area, a strange alternating sequence. The latter two areas are the posterior and anterior parts of the hypothalamus (**Fig. 6-2**).

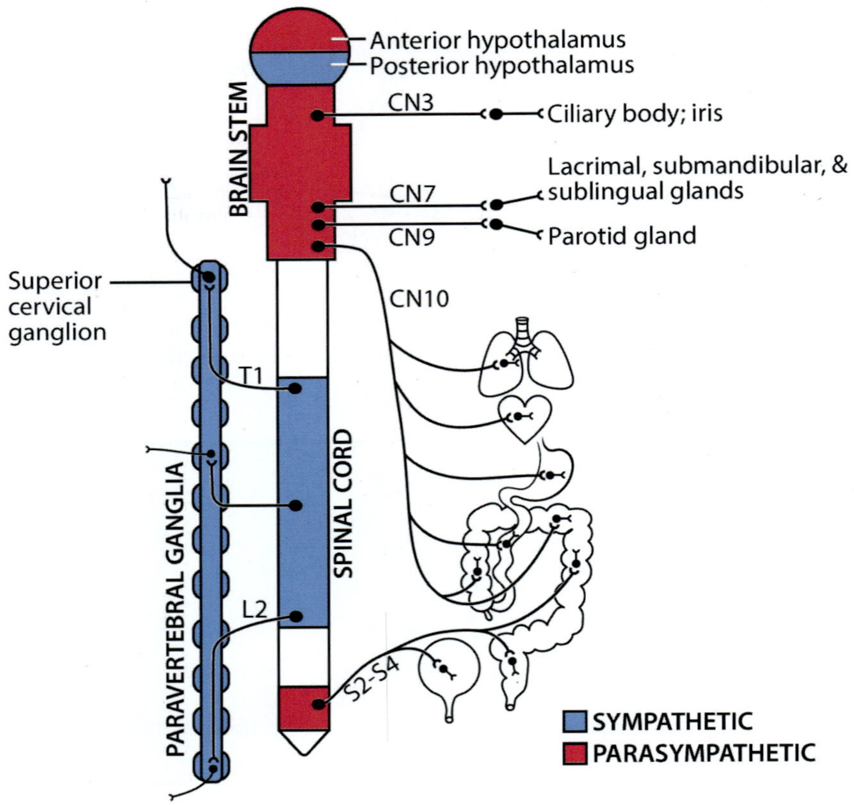


*Figure 6-2* *Schematic view of the autonomic nervous system.*

The hypothalamus, a structure about the size of a thumbnail, is the master control for the autonomic system. Stimulation or lesions result not in isolated smooth muscle, cardiac muscle, or glandular effects but in organized actions involving these systems, e.g., in the fear or rage reaction of the flight-or-fight response, in increased and decreased appetite, altered sexual functioning, and control of body temperature. For instance, stimulation of the posterior hypothalamus may result in conservation of body heat and an increase in body temperature owing to constriction of cutaneous blood vessels.

Many circuits connect the hypothalamus with various areas of the cerebral cortex, brain stem and thalamus. **Figure 6-4** shows the reverberating **Papez circuit** believed to be involved in the emotional content of conscious thought processes and in memory. It provides intercommunication between hippocampus, hypothalamus, thalamus and cerebral cortex. Note the input of the olfactory system, which also plays a role in emotion. This is evident if you have ever seen two dogs sniffing one another or noted the prominence of the perfume industry in major department stores. In the **Klüver-Bucy syndrome**, there are lesions of the amygdala, resulting in docile behavior, hypersexuality, compulsive attentiveness to detail, and, with injury to nearby areas, visual agnosia (inability to recognize objects visually).

| FIGURE 6-3. SYMPATHETIC AND PARASYMPATHETIC FUNCTIONS | | |
|---|---|---|
| **STRUCTURE** | **SYMPATHETIC FUNCTION** | **PARASYMPATHETIC FUNCTION** |
| **Eye** | • Dilates pupil (mydriasis)<br>• No significant effect on ciliary muscle | • Contracts pupil (miosis)<br>• Contracts ciliary muscle (accommodation) |
| **Lacrimal gland** | No significant effect | Stimulates secretion |
| **Salivary glands** | Stimulates viscous secretion | Stimulates watery secretion |
| **Sweat glands** | Stimulates secretion (cholinergic fibers) | No significant effect |
| **Heart**<br>Rate<br>Force of ventricular contraction | <br>Increases heart rate<br>Increases force | <br>Decreases heart rate<br>Decreases force |
| **Blood vessels** | • Dilates or constricts cardiac & skeletal muscle vessels*<br>• Constricts skin and digestive system blood vessels | No significant effect |
| **Lungs** | Dilates bronchial tubes | • Constricts bronchial tubes<br>• Stimulates bronchial gland secretion |
| **Gastrointestinal tract** | Inhibits motility and secretion | Stimulates motility and secretion |
| **GI sphincters** | Contracts | Relaxes |
| **Adrenal medulla** | Stimulates secretion of adrenaline (cholinergic fibers) | No significant effect |
| **Urinary bladder** | Relaxes (minimal) | Contracts |
| **Sex organs** | Ejaculation | Erection** |
| **Liver** | Stimulates gluconeogenesis & glycogenolysis | |
| **Fat** | Stimulates lipolysis | |
| **Kidney** | Stimulates renin release | |

*Stimulation of beta-2 receptors *dilates* cardiac and skeletal muscle vessels, whereas stimulation of alpha-1 receptors *constricts*. Most dilation of cardiac and skeletal vessels, though, may be due to nonautonomic, local tissue *autoregulatory* responses to lack of oxygen.
**Parasympathetic = erection, since parasympathetic is a longer word.

In **Wernicke's syndrome**, which occurs in patients who are alcoholic and undernourished, there is paralysis of eye movements, ataxic gait and disturbances in the state of consciousness associated with hemorrhages in the hypothalamus and other regions.

**Korsakoff's syndrome** also occurs in alcoholic patients and consists of memory loss, confusion and confabulation associated with lesions in the mammillary bodies and associated areas.

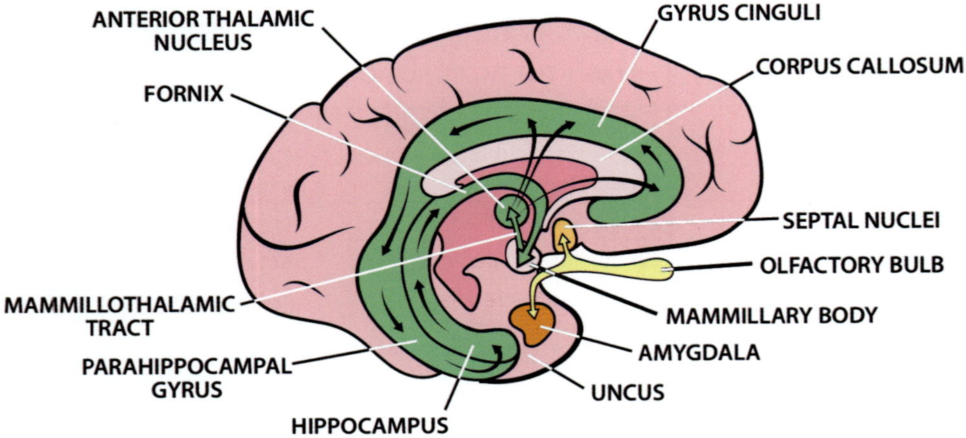


***Figure 6-4*** *The Papez circuit (green shaded areas). The labeled structures as a whole are referred to as the limbic system. The hippocampus, among other things, is involved in the storage of short-term memory. (Modified from Clark, R.G.,* Manter & Gatz's Esssentials of Clinical Neuroanatomy & Neurophysiology, *F.A. Davis Co., Phila., 1975).*

The hypothalamus lies close to the pituitary gland. A disorder of one structure may affect the other. **Figure 6-5** shows the major hypothalamopituitary connections. Note that nerve fibers from the *paraventricular* and *supraoptic nuclei* of the hypothalamus connect with the posterior pituitary. These nuclei secrete the hormones *oxytocin* and *antidiuretic hormone* (*vasopressin*). These hormones are synthesized and transported in neurons and then released at the ends of the nerve terminals in the posterior pituitary.

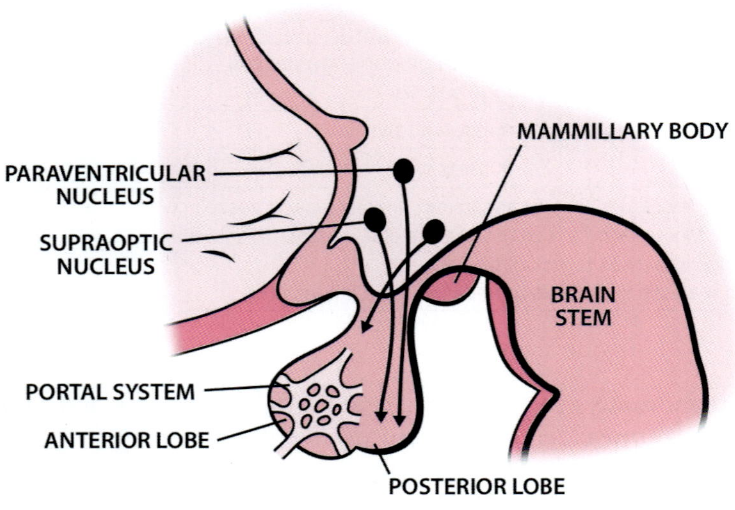


***Figure 6-5*** *The connections between the hypothalamus and pituitary gland.*

The anterior pituitary contains no neuronal connections. Instead, *releasing factors* are produced in the hypothalamus; they are released into the portal circulation and then transported to the anterior pituitary. There, they stimulate cells in the anterior pituitary to secrete various hormones, including adrenocorticotrophic hormone, thyrotrophic hormone, somatotrophic hormone, follicle-stimulating hormone and luteinizing hormone.

Disorders of the autonomic system include:

1. **Riley-Day syndrome** (familial dysautonomia), a disease associated with degenerative changes in the central nervous system and the peripheral autonomic system. Symptoms include decreased lacrimation, transient skin blotching, attacks of hypertension, episodes of hyperpyrexia and vomiting, impairment of taste discrimination, relative insensitivity to pain, and emotional instability.
2. **Adiposogenital syndrome**, characterized by obesity and retarded development of secondary sexual characteristics, sometimes associated with lesions in the hypothalamus
3. **Precocious puberty** may result from hypothalamic tumors.
4. **The common cold**. Temperature elevation is apparently the consequence of an influence on hypothalamic functioning.
5. Tumors of the pituitary may have a destructive effect on the pituitary gland and hypothalamus by direct extension, e.g., chromophobe adenoma and craniopharyngioma are generally nonsecretory tumors. If the tumor contains functioning glandular tissue e.g., acidophilic or basophilic adenoma, there may be the opposite effect of hypersecretion of pituitary hormones.
6. **Diabetes insipidus.** Vasopressin (antidiuretic hormone) enhances the reuptake of water in the kidney. Interference with its production, as by an invading tumor, leads to diabetes insipidus, characterized by excessive production of urine and excessive thirst (up to 20 liters imbibed daily).
7. **Horner's syndrome**. Interruption of the cervical sympathetic nerves (or in some cases their central origins in the spinal cord and brain stem) leads to ptosis, miosis, and anhydrosis (decreased sweating) on the involved side of the face. Sometimes this is the result of a tumor of the apex of the lung (*Pancoast tumor*) that interrupts the fibers as they course from the superior cervical ganglion (the most rostral ganglion in the sympathetic chain) to the carotid artery on their way to the orbit.

   Surgical procedures were historically performed to interrupt the sympathetic innervation of the lower extremities in order to increase circulation in cases of vascular insufficiency.
8. **Hirschsprung's megacolon**—Congenital absence of parasympathetic ganglion cells in the wall of the colon, resulting in poor colonic motility and a dilated colon.
9. **Multiple System Atrophy** is a condition, usually in men over 50 years old, that resembles Parkinson's disease (slowness, stiffness, mask-like facies, pill-rolling tremor) along with autonomic symptoms (fainting when standing up, loss of bowel/bladder control, impotence, decreased sweating, nausea, and digestive problems).
10. Most autonomic problems are medication side effects.

# 7

# Cerebellum, Basal Ganglia, and Thalamus

Clinically, it is not very important to know the complex internal connections of the thalamus, cerebellum and basal ganglia, and these will not be emphasized.

## The Thalamus

The thalamus is a sensory relay and integrative center connecting with many areas of the brain including the cerebral cortex, basal ganglia, hypothalamus, and brain stem. It is capable of perceiving pain but not of accurate localization. For instance, patients with tumors of the thalamus may experience the "thalamic pain syndrome"—a vague sense of pain without the ability to accurately localize it. Sensory fibers, ascending through the brain stem, synapse in the thalamus and are then relayed to the cerebral cortex via the internal capsule. Motor fibers descending from the cerebral cortex pass to the brain stem via the internal capsule without synapsing in the thalamus. **Figure 7-1** illustrates the anatomy of this region.

Notable thalamic nuclei include: the ventral posterolateral (VPL) nucleus, a synaptic region for ascending spinal sensory pathways (**Fig. 3-2**); the ventral posteromedial (VPM) nucleus, the synaptic area for the trigeminal lemniscus (**Fig. 4-3**); the anterior thalamic nucleus, which is a part of the Papez circuit (**Fig. 6-4**); the ventral lateral (VL) nucleus, which receives input from the cerebellum (**Fig. 7-2**). There are some 50-60 thalamic nuclei, but from a non-neurosurgical perspective, just knowing the word "thalamus" is sufficient.

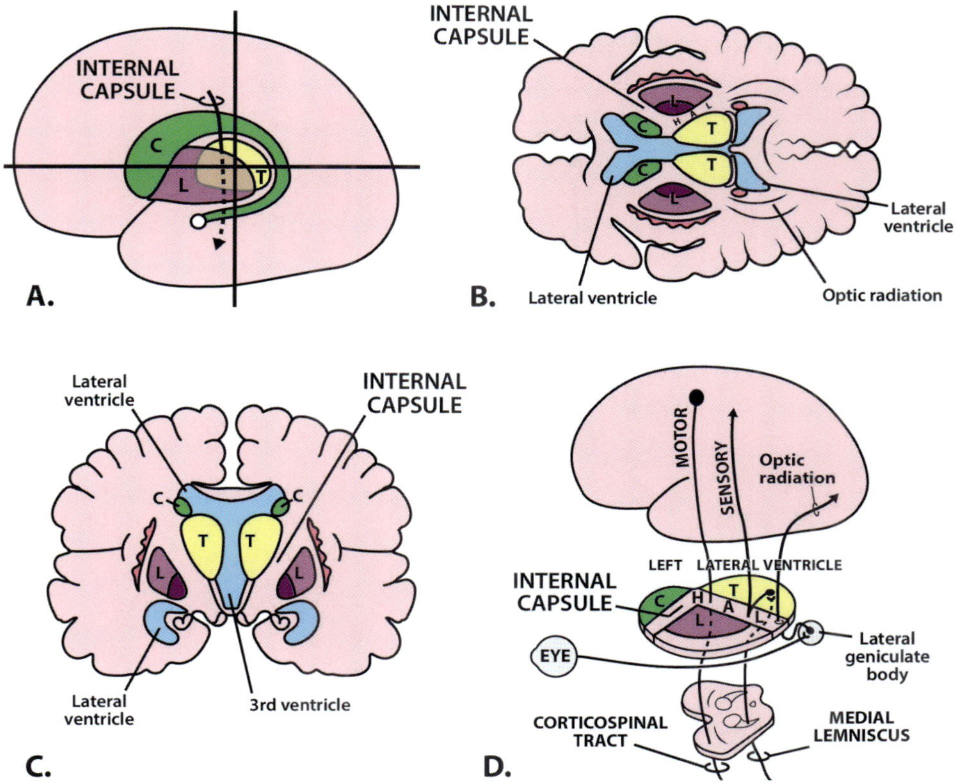


*Figure 7-1* *The internal capsule and its relationship to the caudate nucleus (C), thalamus (T), and lentiform nucleus (L). A. Lateral view. B. Horizontal section at the level indicated in A. C. Cross section at the level indicated in A. D. The course of the major motor and sensory pathways. H, head; A, arm; L, leg.*

The **lentiform nucleus** (the **putamen** plus **globus pallidus**) lies lateral to the internal capsule, and the caudate nucleus and thalamus lie medial. Note in **Figure 7-1D** the distribution of head, arm, and leg fibers in the internal capsule.

## The Cerebellum And Basal Ganglia

Rather than list the multitude of complex cerebellar and basal ganglia connections, it is clinically more important to understand the types of clinical syndromes that may occur in these two systems. In general, cerebellar dysfunction is characterized by awkwardness of intentional movements. Basal ganglia disorders are more characterized by meaningless unintentional movements occurring unexpectedly at rest.

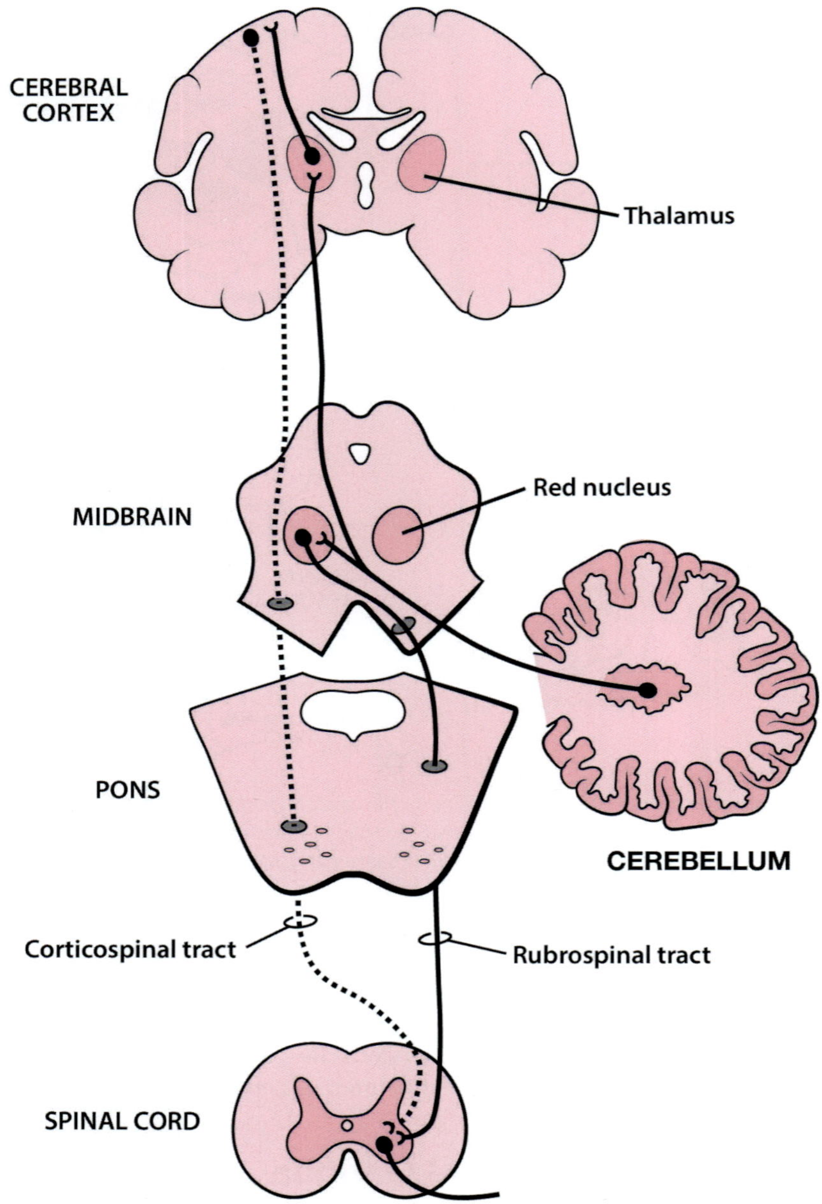


***Figure 7-2*** *The relationship between the cerebellum and the red nucleus (Modified from Clark, R.G.,* Manter & Gatz's Esssentials of Clinical Neuroanatomy & Neurophysiology, *F.A. Davis Co., Phila., 1975).*

## Cerebellar Disorders

1. **Ataxia**—awkwardness of posture and gait; tendency to fall to the same side as the cerebellar lesion; poor coordination of movement; overshooting the goal in reaching toward an object (**dysmetria**); inability to perform rapid alternating movements (**dysdiadochokinesia**), such as finger tapping; **scanning speech** due to awkward use of speech muscles, resulting in irregularly spaced sounds
2. Decreased tendon reflexes on the affected side
3. **Asthenia**—muscles tire more easily than normal and are not relieved by rest.
4. **Tremor**—usually an intention tremor (evident during purposeful movements). **Titubation** is a rhythmic oscillation of the head or trunk, typically seen when the person is sitting or standing.
5. **Nystagmus**

## Basal Ganglia Disorders

1. **Parkinson's disease**—rigidity; slowness; resting tremor; mask-like facies; shuffling gait, associated with degeneration in the basal ganglia and midbrain substantia nigra gray matter.
2. **Chorea**—sudden jerky and purposeless movements (e.g., **Sydenham's chorea** found in rheumatic fever and Huntington's chorea, an inherited disorder).
3. **Athetosis**—slow writhing, snake-like movements, especially of the fingers and wrists.
4. **Hemiballismus**—a sudden wild flail-like movement of one arm.

# 8

# Cerebral Cortex

Lesions to the nervous system may lead to simple or complex levels of dysfunction depending upon the area involved. For instance, if one asks a patient to put on a polo shirt and their left brachial plexus is damaged, they will only use the right arm, as the left arm is paralyzed. The cerebellum and basal ganglia represent a step further in levels of functioning. With a cerebellar lesion, the patient may perform the act awkwardly, e.g. overshooting the mark, or with tremor. With basal ganglia lesions there may be unexpected, unplanned totally irrelevant movements, beyond the realm of awkwardness, e.g., a sudden flail-like movement. In the cerebral cortex, unless the lesion is in the primary motor area wherein paralysis may result, a higher level of dysfunction may be found, e.g., trying to get the head into the sleeve or trying other inadequate orientations.

In speech, a lesion of CN10 may result in hoarseness (laryngeal dysfunction). When cranial nerves 10, 12, or 7 are involved, there may be difficulty with the "KLM" sounds: i.e., the sounds "Kuh, Kuh, Kuh" test the soft palate (CN10), "LA, LA, LA," the tongue (CN12) and "MI, MI, MI" the lips (CN7). With lesions in the speech areas of the cerebral cortex, the deficit may involve higher levels of speech organization—the deletion of words or inclusion of excessive or inappropriate words. In psychiatric disturbances the level of dysfunction is even higher with abnormalities in the entire pattern of thought organization.

It is similar for the sensory pathways. Simple anesthesia may result from lesions between the primary sensory cortex and the body periphery. In other brain areas, the patient may have difficulty in comprehending the incoming information. For instance, a lesion to the optic tract results in homonymous hemianopia (**Fig. 5-1E**). In lesions to cortical areas 18 and 19 the patient sees but may not recognize what he is looking at.

Complex cerebral receptive disabilities are called **agnosias**. Complex cerebral motor disabilities are **apraxias**. Often the two are difficult to distinguish.

When language function is involved, the disabilities are termed **aphasias**. Aphasia may be receptive (i.e., reading, listening) or motor (i.e., writing, talking). For aphasia to occur, the lesion must be in the dominant hemisphere, which is the left hemisphere in right-handed people and in many (but not all) left-handed people.

The orange shaded area in **Figure 8-1** indicates the region of the cerebral cortex involved with aphasia. Subdivisions of this area are logical. Lesions in the anterior part of this area, near the motor cortex, tend to result in expressive aphasia. Lesions more posterior, near the auditory and visual cortex, result in receptive aphasia. Lesions nearer the visual cortex result in inability to read (**alexia**). Lesions near the auditory cortex result in inability to understand speech.

Difficulty in talking may result from either anterior or posterior lesions. Following lesions in the more anterior regions of the aphasic zone, speech disturbances tend to be nonfluent; the patient omits nouns and connector words like *but*, *or*, and *and*. In the more posterior regions. his words are plentiful or even excessive, but he crams into his speech inappropriate word substitutes, circumlocutions and neologisms—a word salad. Presumably, this is because the ability to speak also depends on the ability to understand what one is saying. Thus, if the aphasic area near the auditory cortex is involved, this will also result in a defect in speech.

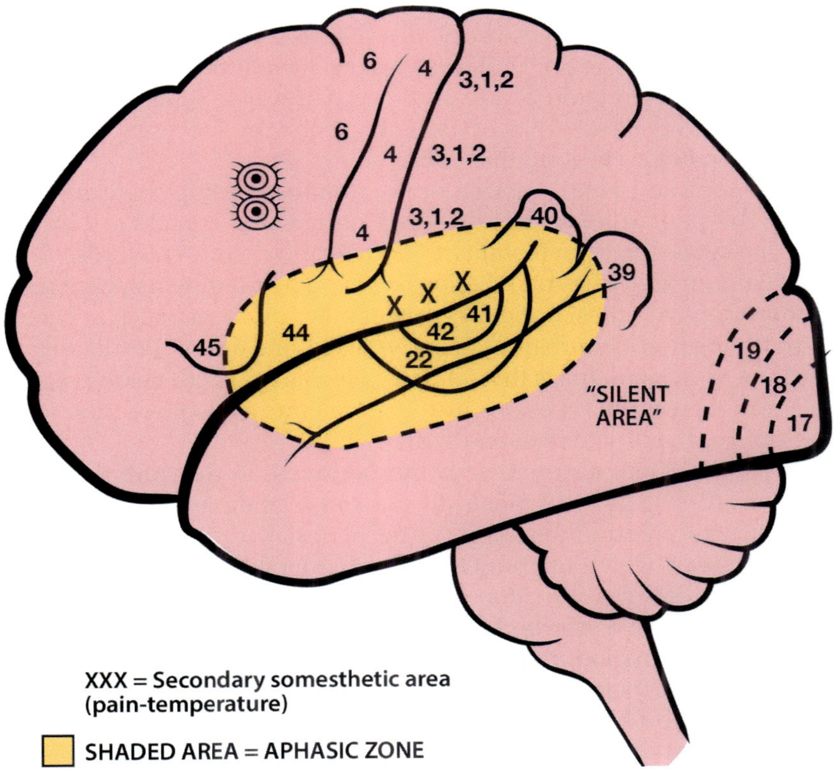


*Figure 8-1 Major regions of the cerebrum.*

Lesions to corresponding areas of the non-dominant hemisphere do not result in aphasia, but rather in visual or auditory inattention to the left environment or to general unawareness of the concept of "left." The patient may deny they have any neurological deficit despite a dense hemiplegia and left visual field defect.

Specific cerebral cortical regions and the effects of lesions are listed below.

- Area 4 (the primary motor area). Lesions result in initial flaccid paralysis followed in several months by partial recovery of function and a possible Babinski reflex; spasticity and increased deep tendon reflexes may occur if area 6 (the supplemental motor area) is included.
- Lesions to area 8 (the frontal eye fields) result in difficulty in voluntarily moving the eyes to the opposite side.
- Areas of the frontal cortex rostral to the motor areas are involved in complex behavioral activities. Lesions result in changes in judgment, abstract thinking, tactfulness, and foresight. Symptoms may include irresponsibility in dealing with daily affairs, vulgar speech, and clownish behavior.
- Areas 44, 45 (Broca's speech area). The patient with a lesion in this area experiences motor aphasia, but only when the dominant hemisphere is involved. The patient knows what they want to say but speech is slow, deleting many prepositions and nouns.
- Areas 3, 1, 2 (primary somesthetic area). Lesions produce contralateral impairment of touch, pressure, and proprioception. Pain sensation will be impaired if the lesion lies in the secondary somesthetic sensory area (**Fig. 8-1**) which receives pain information.
- Areas 41, 42 (auditory area). Unilateral lesions have little effect on hearing owing to the bilateral representation of the auditory pathways. Significant auditory defects generally involve either CN8 or its entry point in the brain stem, for bilateral representation begins beyond this point.
- Area 22 (Wernicke's area). Lesions in the dominant hemisphere result in auditory aphasia. The patient hears but does not understand, speaking but unknowingly making mistakes due to an inability to understand their own words.
- Area 40 (supramarginal gyrus). Lesions in the dominant hemisphere result in tactile and proprioceptive agnosia, and a variety of other problems, such as confusion in left-right discrimination, disturbances of body-image, and apraxia, by cutting off impulses to and from association tracts that interconnect this area with nearby regions.
- Area 39 (angular gyrus). Lesions in the dominant hemisphere may result in alexia and agraphia (inability to read and write).
- Areas 17, 18, 19. Total destruction causes blindness in the contralateral visual field. Lesions to areas 18 and 19 alone do not cause blindness but rather difficulty in recognizing and identifying objects (visual agnosia).
- The "silent area," which might not produce immediately obvious symptoms when damaged, is believed to function in memory storage and processing of visual and auditory information and is implicated in hallucinations and dreams. Epileptic attacks originating in this region may be associated with amnesia, auditory hallucinations, and the deja vu phenomenon.
- The basal nucleus of Meynert lies in the base of the frontal lobe just lateral to the optic chiasm. Degeneration of this nucleus is associated with the dementia of Alzheimer's disease.

# 9

# Neurotransmitters

Neurotransmitters are chemicals that are released from the ends of nerve cell axons and interact with postsynaptic cell receptors, either stimulating or inhibiting the firing of nerve or other cells. Decreases or increases in neurotransmitter function can significantly influence nervous system activity.

While some neurotransmitters are referred to as "inhibitory" or "excitatory," this classification is a bit misleading, since neurotransmitters are neither intrinsically inhibitory nor excitatory. Their action depends on their receptors; some kinds of receptors can be stimulated, while others can be inhibited by the same neurotransmitter. Thus, a given neurotransmitter can be both inhibitory and excitatory, depending on the receptor. Moreover, even if a neurotransmitter excites a receptor and causes postsynaptic nerve cell firing, the firing cell may inhibit the next neuron in the line, and the neurotransmitter has a net inhibitory effect.

Numerous neurotransmitters are scattered throughout the nervous system, and, while some may be more confined to particular regions or nuclei, knowing the anatomy of these regions and nuclei is not as important as understanding the effects of a general decline or increase of the neurotransmitter, which may be more widespread than in a single isolated area. Thus, it is generally more important to know the effects of a general decline or increase in availability or function of a particular neurotransmitter than its particular location in the brain. Since neurotransmitters are widespread in the brain, affecting a neurotransmitter may have widespread effects, whether good or bad.

Too *much* neurotransmission can be caused by drugs, heredity, environmental factors (e.g., diet, stress, exercise, toxins, sleep disturbances) or certain neurologic diseases that either increase the release of neurotransmitters, inhibit degradation of neurotransmitters, or act as agonists (mimics) at postsynaptic receptors. Too *little* neurotransmission can be caused by drugs, heredity, age, environmental factors, and certain neurologic diseases that decrease neurotransmitter activity. Medications that alter neurotransmitter levels are used in the treatment of certain neurologic diseases.

The neurotransmitter *dopamine,* found in various regions of the brain, including the substantia nigra of the midbrain, is low in Parkinson's disease and is believed to be high in schizophrenia. Antipsychotic drugs may therefore produce Parkinsonism as a side effect, due to their decrease of dopamine transmission.

*Acetylcholine* and *norepinephrine* are the main neurotransmitters in the peripheral nervous system, which includes the cranial nerves, spinal nerves, and the autonomic nervous system. Acetylcholine (Ach), in addition to its autonomic function, stimulates receptors at the neuromuscular junction of skeletal muscles, enabling muscle contraction. Myasthenia gravis is an autoimmune disease where antibodies block skeletal muscle Ach receptors in skeletal muscles, resulting in muscle weakness. It is treated with *physostigmine,* an anticholinesterase, which prevents the breakdown of Ach, thereby keeping more Ach around. *Curare,* the "arrow poison," blocks the action of Ach at the neuromuscular junction, resulting in paralysis.

Acetylcholine is an important transmitter in the central nervous system as well, where it may have both excitatory and inhibitor receptors and is important in memory. Alzheimer's disease may be associated with a deficiency of acetylcholine in certain areas of the brain and is treated with acetylcholinesterase inhibitors.

The monoamines *serotonin, norepinephrine,* and *dopamine,* when deficient, are believed important in the genesis of depression. Thus, drugs to help combat these disorders include:

- Selective serotonin reuptake inhibitors (SSRIs), e.g., *Prozac, Lexapro*
- Norepinephrine reuptake inhibitors (NRIs), e.g., *Strattera*
- Combined serotonin-norepinephrine reuptake inhibitors (SNRIs), such as the tricyclic antidepressant *Elavil* and newer drugs such as *Effexor* and *Cymbalta*
- Combined dopamine-norepinephrine uptake inhibitors, e.g., *Wellbutrin*
- Monoamine oxidase inhibitors (MAOIs), e.g., *Nardil, Parnate.* MAO is a family of enzymes that break down monoamines, such as serotonin, norepinephrine, and dopamine, so MAO inhibitors can be useful in treating depression.

*Dopamine* and *amphetamine* excess produce a feeling of increased energy, less need for sleep, and an accelerated sense of time; they can also lead to hallucinations and paranoid thinking. Mania (a hyperexcited mood and energy state) is believed related to overactivity of certain dopamine receptors. *Cocaine* increases dopaminergic activity. *Marijuana* can reduce dopaminergic activity and slows the feeling of subjective time.

Stimulant drugs that increase dopamine in the brain (e.g., *Ritalin*) or have amphetamine-like effects (e.g., *Adderall*) have been useful in treating ADHD (Attention Deficit Hyperactivity Disorder), enabling patients to increase their focus.

*Phenylethylamine* (PEA) is a neurotransmitter in the brain that is associated with sexual attraction and excitement, peaking in orgasm and ovulation. It releases norepinephrine and dopamine. PEA is found in chocolate, but (unfortunately) is quickly metabolized when taken orally so that significant amounts do not reach the brain.

*Glycine* is an inhibitory transmitter. Strychnine poison is a glycine antagonist; it binds to the glycine receptor, resulting in spinal hyperexcitability, with severe muscle spasms, convulsions, and death.

*Gamma-aminobutyric acid (GABA*; "N**A**ture's V**A**lium") is an inhi**B**itory amino acid neurotransmitter (in 90% of instances). Benzodiazepines and barbiturates enhance the actions of certain GABA receptors and are used as sedatives to treat anxiety, seizures, and the hyperactive muscle action of people with Huntington's disease.

*GluTamaTe (glutamic acid)* is the main exci**T**a**T**ory neurotransmitter in the brain. Glutamate excitotoxicity has been implicated in the development of Huntington's chorea, Alzheimer's Disease, and amyotrophic lateral sclerosis (ALS). Alertness due to caffeine ingestion may be related to its effect on increasing glutamate levels in the brain.

*Opioids*. Opioid receptors are found in a number of areas in the nervous system. *Endorphins*, *enkephalins*, and *dynorphins* are natural body chemicals that interact with opiate receptors. They are powerful natural pain relievers. *Opium* and *morphine* mimic the natural opioids by binding to opioid receptors, thereby reducing pain. Opioid overdose can be treated with antagonists to opioid receptors, such as *naloxone (Narcan)*.

*Substance **P*** and *CGR**P*** (Calcitonin Gene-Related Peptide) are widespread neurotransmitters that among other things, are involved in the production of **P**ain, as in migraine. Medications that reduce levels of substance P and CGRP can be used as analgesics.

*Melatonin*, produced mainly in the pineal gland, promotes sleep and is administered in the treatment of certain sleep disorders.

*Histamine*, primarily synthesized and stored in tissue mast cells and basophils and plays an important role in inflammation, is also produced in brain stem neurons, where it plays a role in arousal, mood, and cognitive function. *Pitolisant* (a brain histamine H3 receptor antagonist) may be administered in treating narcolepsy, a sleep disorder.

Following injury, severed axons of the peripheral nervous system can regenerate, growing back to their targets at a rate of about 1-2 mm/day. The central nervous system, though, does not regenerate well, but motor and sensory function can improve through the brain's self-modification of alternative neural pathways and the use of a variety of mechanical and digital devices. Another approach is to pharmacologically enhance neurotransmitter activity.

# 10

# *Principles of Neurologic Localization*

The first step in neurologic evaluation is determining *where* the problem lies, then *what* the problem is. Does the problem lie in the cerebral cortex, internal capsule, cerebellum, basal ganglia, brain stem, spinal cord, peripheral nerve, or elsewhere?

*Malingering Versus Functional Neurologic Disorder (FND)*

Malingering is the deliberate faking or exaggeration of symptoms for external gain. However, many patients present with legitimate neurological symptoms—such as weakness, seizures, or sensory loss—that do not follow typical anatomical patterns and are not confirmed by lab tests. These patients are not "faking" or "psychological" in the traditional sense (the old terms were "hysteria/conversion disorder"). Modern medicine recognizes these symptoms as part of Functional Neurological Disorder (FND)—a real, brain-based condition affecting nervous system function without structural damage. FND affects up to 16% of neurology outpatients and includes functional weakness, functional seizures, functional movement disorders, and functional sensory symptoms.

**Clues Suggesting Malingering:**

- Clear secondary gain (e.g., lawsuit, disability claim, criminal defense)
- Overly dramatic or inconsistent presentation
- Symptoms worsen when observed and improve when unobserved.
- Refusal of diagnostic tests or treatment, especially when results could challenge their claims

- Symptoms don't make anatomical sense.
- "Glove and stocking" numbness (unless diabetic)
- Weakness that "gives way": The limb resists briefly, then suddenly gives way—unlike organic motor loss.
- Reflexes before you tap them

**Signs Suggesting Functional Neurological Disorder (FND):**

- Tremor Entrainment Test: A functional tremor may change frequency or stop when the patient is asked to tap a rhythm with the opposite hand, indicating distractibility.
- Midline-Splitting Sensory Loss: Sensory loss that stops exactly at the body's midline, inconsistent with known neuroanatomy.
- Inconsistent Speech Deficits: Speech abnormalities such as whispering or stuttering that vary with attention or normalize during distraction.
- Normal Movement During Automatic Tasks: The patient may be unable to move a limb on command but use it spontaneously during unguarded movements (e.g., scratching, catching).
- Eyes Tightly Shut During Seizure-like Events: Common in psychogenic non-epileptic seizures, unlike true epileptic seizures where the eyes are usually open and unresponsive. There may also be uncharacteristic side-to-side head movements in FND-type seizures, gradual onset and offset, and a normal EEG during events.
- Rapid Recovery Post-Event: Absence of postictal confusion, fatigue, or injury following a seizure-like episode—unlike true epileptic seizures.
- Hoover's Sign: The examiner places a hand under the heel of the "weak" leg while asking the patient to flex the opposite hip against resistance. Normally, flexing one hip automatically produces extension of the opposite hip.
  - In organic paralysis: The weak leg does not extend because the motor pathway is truly impaired.
  - In malingering (faking): The weak leg also does not extend, because the patient consciously withholds effort.
  - In FND: The weak leg extends normally during contralateral hip flexion, even though it cannot extend on direct testing. This inconsistency demonstrates intact motor pathways but impaired voluntary control.

**There are signs that cannot be faked:**

- Significant asymmetry in the pupillary light reflex
- Abnormal retinal appearance
- Ocular divergence
- Marked nystagmus
- Muscle atrophy and fasciculation
- Babinski reflex and asymmetric reflexes
- Multiple complex signs and symptoms that can be explained by a single small lesion also suggest an organic disease.

The detection of symptomatic signs inconsistent with neuroanatomy does not necessarily mean that the patient's entire condition is non-neuroanatomical. For example, a patient may have a real neuroanatomical headache and also a projection of pain down the same side of the body, which is not likely neuroanatomically, since one side of the brain connects with the opposite body.

Distinguishing FND from malingering can be difficult. Since FND involves involuntary symptoms without conscious deception, patients should be treated with empathy and validation. Explain that the symptoms are real and not "all in your head," that the condition is common and treatable. These patients benefit from specialized treatment focusing on restoring normal function. Early recognition and appropriate referral lead to good outcomes.

Although malingering involves intentional deception, accusations should only be made with great caution and thorough documentation, often with input from a neuropsychologist or forensic specialist.

***Is There a Lesion in the Cerebral Cortex?***

- Lesions in the **cerebral cortex** and **internal capsule** both result in contralateral sensory and motor defects, i.e., weakness or sensory loss on the opposite side. It may be difficult to differentiate a lesion in the cerebral cortex from one in the internal capsule. The presence of higher-level dysfunction is more consistent with a cerebral cortex lesion. This may include confusion, memory loss, an **agnosia** (complex receptive disability, e.g., loss of ability to understand what one is reading while retaining the ability to see), **apraxia** (complex motor disability, such as putting on one's pants backwards), or **aphasia** (complex speech disturbance, as opposed to simple hoarseness or monotone).
- A lesion to the internal capsule or cerebral cortex will not significantly affect most cranial nerve nuclei, because of *bilateral innervation*. That is, most cranial nerve nuclei receive bilateral innervation from the cerebral cortex. Thus, if one side of the cerebrum or internal capsule is injured, the other side takes over function. There are a few key cranial motor and sensory deficits, though, that may occur with a cerebral lesion:

   a. Paralysis of the opposite lower face (CN7) and, in some patients, weakness of the opposite side of the tongue (CN12) (**Fig. 4-4**).
   b. Sensation loss to the entire opposite face (CN5).
   c. Whereas there is no paralysis of the opposite eye muscles, there may be inability of either eye to look conjugately toward the opposite side. The eyes will passively "look toward the lesion."
   d. Rather than blindness in the opposite eye, the individual may have loss of vision affecting the ability of either eye to see the opposite visual field.

If other cranial nerves show a deficit, it implies that the lesion lies either within the cranial nerve itself or in the nucleus of the nerve within the brain stem, not in the internal capsule or cerebral cortex. If there is bilateral involvement of the other cranial nerves, there may be a bilateral cerebral cortex or bilateral internal capsule lesion (**pseudobulbar palsy**).

### Is There a Cerebellar or Basal Ganglia Lesion?

**Cerebellar** and **basal ganglia** lesions both result in motor problems, specifically in aberrations in the quality of coordinated movements, as opposed to paralysis. Cerebellar dysfunction is characterized by awkwardness of intentional movements (e.g., intention tremor, ataxia) with no awkwardness at rest. Basal ganglia disorders are more characterized by unintentional movements at rest (e.g., resting tremor, chorea, athetosis, hemiballismus).

### Is There a Brain Stem Lesion?

- The presence of cranial nerve dysfunction (except for the distal extensions of the vagus nerve) confirms that the lesion lies somewhere above the level of the foramen magnum.
- If a cranial nerve deficit is on one side, combined with a contralateral extremity defect (e.g., right facial paralysis and left hemiplegia), the patient likely has a brain stem lesion. A cerebral cortex lesion would have presented with all deficits on the opposite side (e.g., left lower facial paralysis and left hemiplegia).
- The lesion localizes more accurately within the brain stem if any of the following unilateral cranial nerve deficits are noted *along with* the contralateral extremity defects:

1. CN3: Dilated pupil, eye down and out, weakness of eye adduction (**midbrain**)
2. CN4: Cannot move the eye down (**midbrain**)
3. CN5: CN5 dermatome sensory deficit or masseter motor weakness (**pons or medulla)**
4. CN6: Cannot move the eye laterally (**pons**)
5. CN7: Paralysis of BOTH upper & lower face on one side (**pons**)
6. CN8: Deafness on one side (**medulla**)
7. CN9, 10: Vocal cord paralysis; swallowing difficulty (**medulla**)
8. CN11: Difficulty raising the shoulder or turning the head (**medulla**)
9. CN12: Atrophy & fasciculations of the tongue (**medulla**)

A cerebral cortex lesion would not cause these problems because of the principle of bilateral innervation of the brain stem, which spares most cranial nerve nuclei.

- A visual problem confined to one eye indicates that the problem lies anterior to the optic chiasm (in the eye or optic nerve), since optic fibers from each side travel with one another posterior to the chiasm.

### Is There a Spinal Cord Lesion?

- Bilateral paralysis and loss of sensation below a sharp cut-off level at some point below the head suggests a spinal cord injury.
- Dissociation of sensory modalities suggests a spinal cord lesion: e.g., loss of pain-temperature sensation in the right leg and loss of proprioception in the left leg. Only at the spinal cord level can a single lesion produce this deficit, since pain-temperature paths cross at the spinal level, but proprioception-stereognosis is uncrossed until reaching the brain stem (**Fig. 3-2**). Both sensory modalities are crossed in the brain stem and higher.
- A knife sticking into the spinal cord should suggest that area as being the lesion site. Sometimes it is just common sense.

### Is There a Peripheral Nerve Lesion?

- Severing a single spinal nerve root commonly results in little if any motor or sensory defect owing to the overlap distribution of adjacent roots. It may be necessary to sever three or more roots to cause a significant motor or sensory defect. *Spinal nerve root* lesions result in *dermatome* sensory deficits that differ from the patchier sensory loss that occur with lesions of the more peripheral extensions of the nerve. (Compare **Fig. 10-1** and **Fig. 10-2**). This is because a peripheral nerve is a mixture of fibers arising from several nerve roots. The dermatome map represents the distribution of individual nerve roots. The patchy peripheral nerve map represents the fact that individual peripheral nerves are composed of mixtures of nerve roots. The same is true for the motor innervation of muscles (**Fig. 10-3**), which are innervated by mixtures of nerve roots.
- While the peripheral nervous system is neatly partitioned along dermatomes, the central nervous system is not. Lesions of sensory tracts within the CNS characteristically present as general defects in an extremity rather than specific dermatome deficits.
- The presence of localized pain suggests a peripheral nerve lesion, since CNS lesions generally cause loss of pain sensation, rather than pain itself. There are exceptions: Pain may also arise from lesions within the CNS from multiple sclerosis, syringomyelia, and stroke (damage to pain-processing pathways). In the rare thalamic pain syndrome, a thalamic lesion may produce vague, difficult-to-localize pain.
- Sensory loss in a glove-and-stocking fashion indicates either a peripheral neuropathy or a nonphysiologic finding.
- When there is weakness in an extremity, peripheral nerve lesions may be distinguished from internal capsule and cerebral cortical lesions by the presence of lower motor neuron signs (atrophy, fasciculations, decreased reflexes), which result from a peripheral nerve lesion (**Fig. 3-4**). LMN signs also help to localize a lesion, depending on which muscle group is affected (**Fig. 10-3**).
- The combination of UMN signs with a spinal dermatome defect suggests a spinal cord lesion involving motor pathways in the spinal cord along with a lesion to the spinal nerve roots,

### Is the Problem Muscular or Neurological?

- Intrinsic muscular weakness can have a more gradual onset if it's due to a chronic condition like myopathy, whereas nerve weakness might appear more suddenly, as seen in nerve injuries or acute neuropathies.
- Nerve weakness often follows a specific pattern depending on the nerve affected, showing weakness in the distribution of that nerve (**Fig. 10-3**). Intrinsic muscular weakness tends to be more generalized within the specific muscles affected.
- Nerve damage can be associated with pain, numbness, or tingling sensations along the path of the nerve, which is not typical of primary muscular disorders. Altered sensation suggests neural involvement; muscular conditions typically don't affect sensation.
- Both muscular and neurological conditions can lead to muscle atrophy, but atrophy tends to occur more rapidly with nerve damage due to denervation.

- Reduced or absent reflexes can indicate nerve damage. Muscular diseases might not significantly affect reflexes until there is severe muscle wasting.
- Neurological pain often is burning, shooting, or electric shock-like, or presents as paresthesias (pins-and-needles) or numbness. Muscular pain is often aching, sore, or cramping, and localized to specific muscles or joints; it does not generally follow a nerve distribution and may be associated with muscle stiffness, swelling, or tenderness to touch.

Diagnostic tests, as described in **Chapters 13** and **14** can further localize and diagnose the problem.

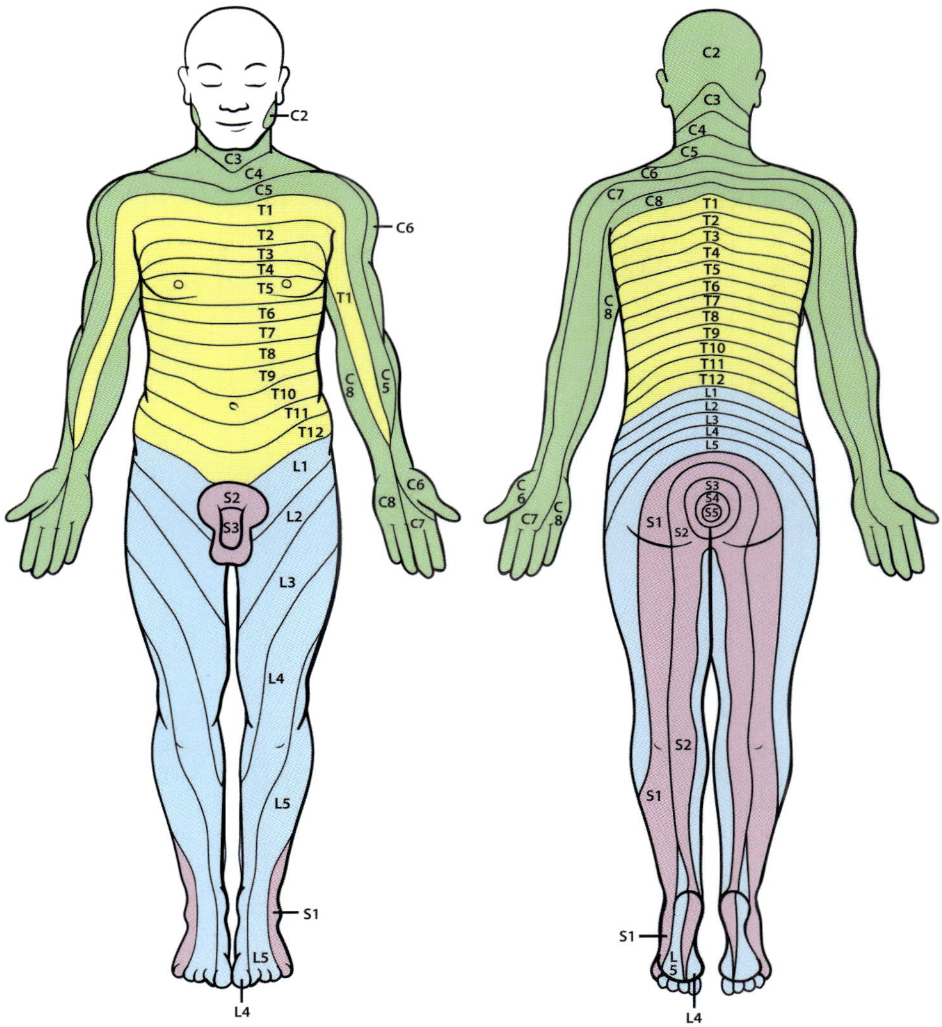


*Figure 10-1* *Dermatome map. C, cervical; T, thoracic; L, lumbar; S, sacral.*

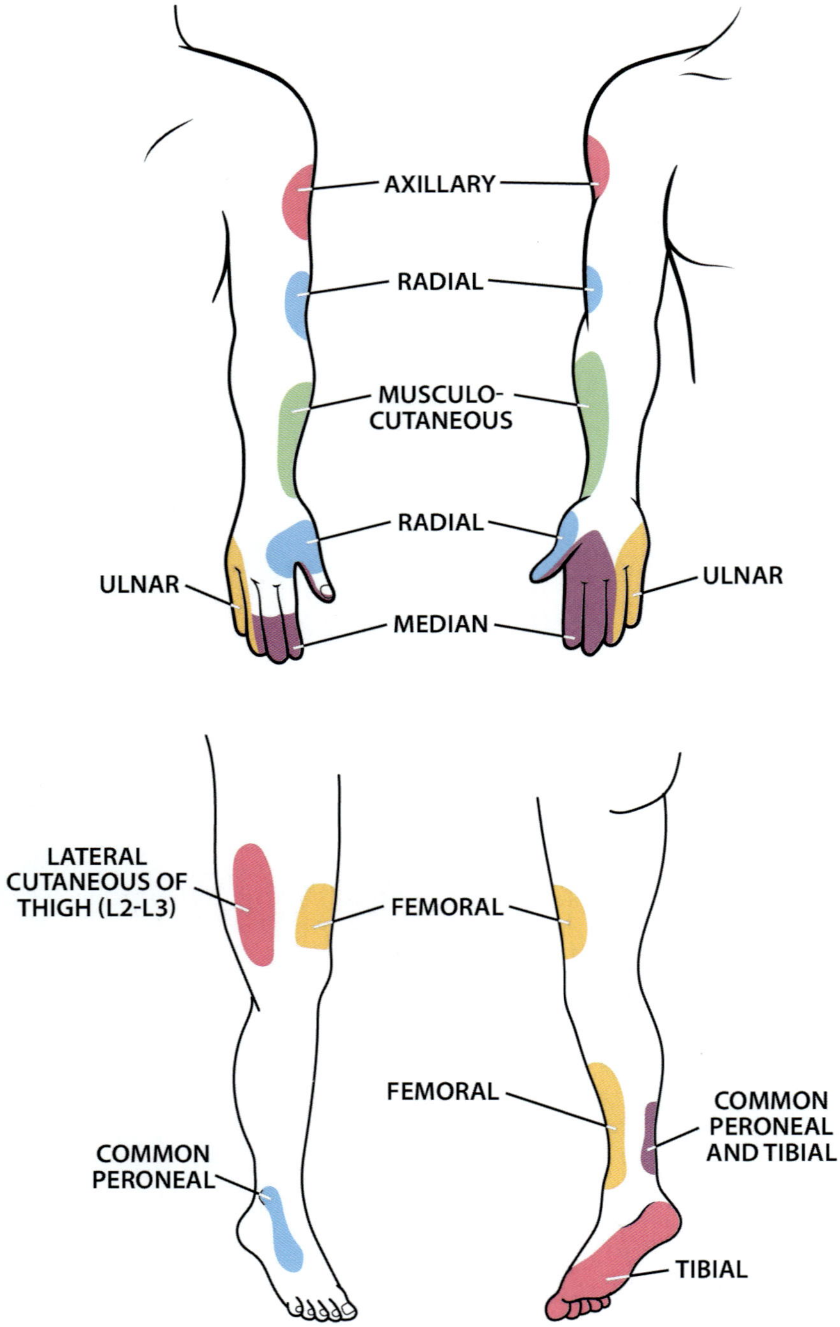


*Figure 10-2* *Sensory defects following peripheral nerve injuries.*

| NERVE | MOTOR FUNCTIONS IMPAIRED WITH INJURY |
|---|---|
| Radial (C5-C8) | Elbow and wrist extension (patient has wrist drop); extension of fingers at metacarpo-phalangeal joints; triceps reflex. |
| Median (C6-T1) | Wrist, thumb, index, and middle finger flexion; thumb opposition, forearm pronation; ability of wrist to bend toward the radial (thumb) side; atrophy of thenar eminence (ball of thumb). |
| Ulnar (C8-T1) | Flexion of wrist, ring and small finger (claw hand); opposition little finger; ability of wrist to bend toward ulnar (small finger) side; adduction and abduction of fingers; atrophy of hypothenar eminence of palm (at base of ring and small fingers). |
| Musculocutaneous(C5-C6) | Elbow flexion (biceps); forearm supination; biceps reflex. |
| Axillary (C5-C6) | Ability to move upper arm outward, forward, or backward (deltoid atrophy). |
| Long thoracic (C5-C7) | Ability to elevate arm above horizontal (patient has winging of scapula.) |
| Femoral (L2-L4) | Knee extension; hip flexion; knee jerk. |
| Obturator (L2-L4) | Hip adduction (patient's leg swings outward when walking). |
| Sciatic (L4-S3) | Knee flexion plus other functions along its branches - the tibial and common peroneal nerves. |
| Tibial (L4-S3) | Foot inversion; ankle plantar flexion; ankle jerk. |
| *Common* peroneal (L4-S2) | Foot eversion; ankle and toes dorsiflexion (patient has high slapping gait owing to foot drop). This nerve is very *commonly* injured. |

***Figure 10-3*** *Motor defects following peripheral nerve injury.*

**Figures 10-4** through **10-9** summarize 24 classic lesions in neurology (arrows indicate which side of the body is symptomatic). Answers at end of figures.

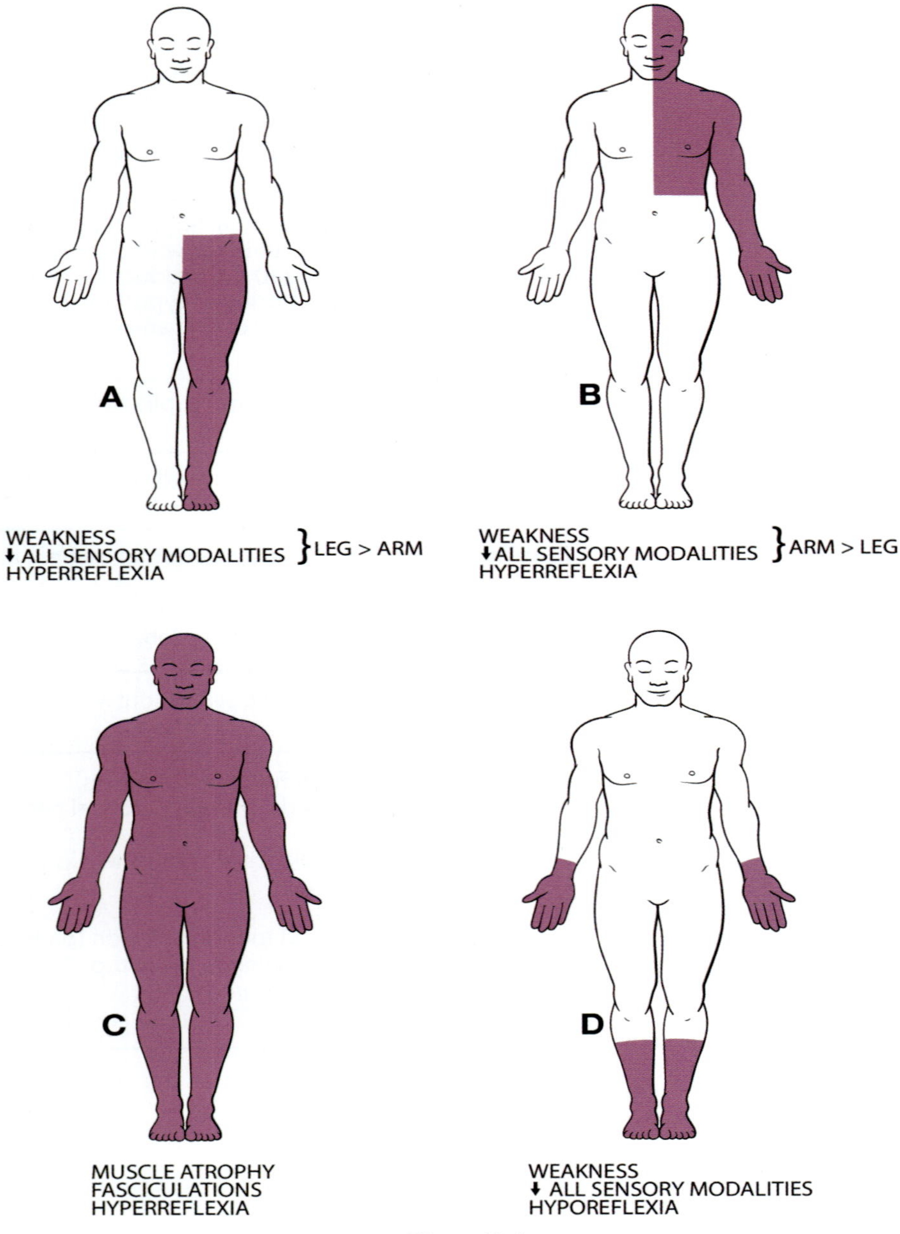


*Figure 10-4*

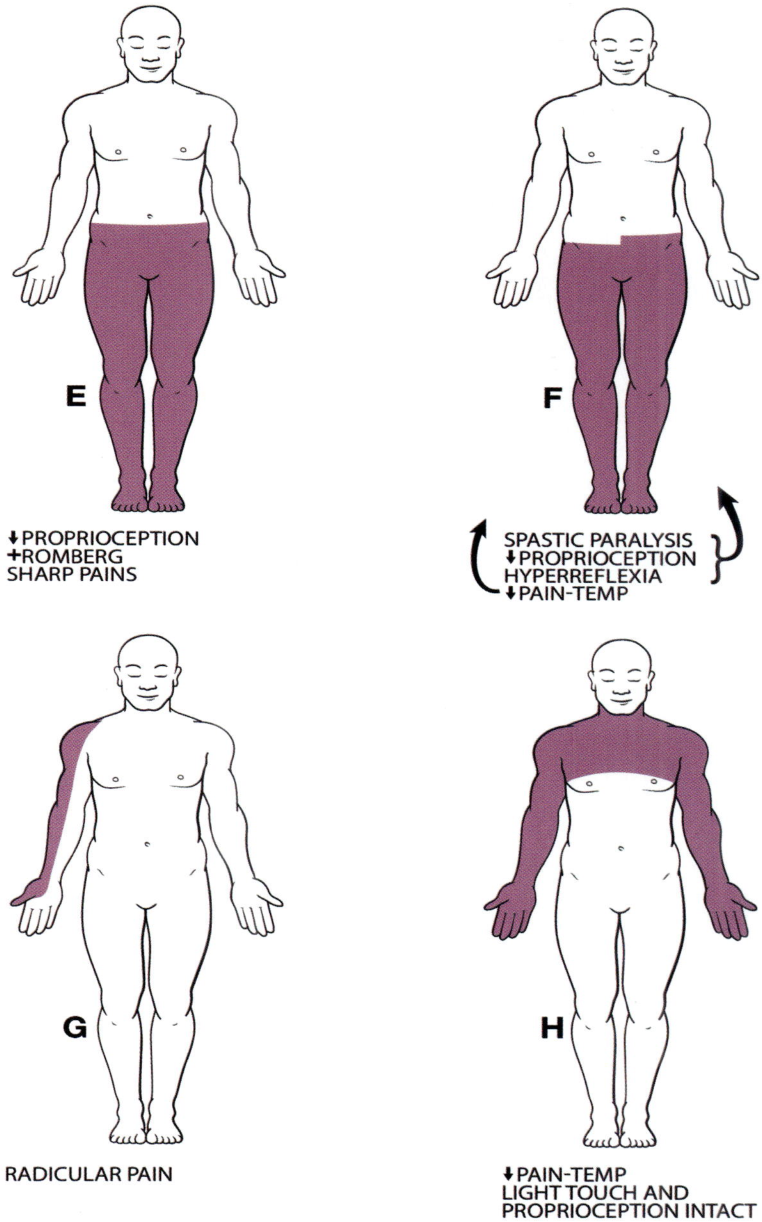
E
↓PROPRIOCEPTION
+ROMBERG
SHARP PAINS
F
SPASTIC PARALYSIS
↓PROPRIOCEPTION
HYPERREFLEXIA
↓PAIN-TEMP
G
RADICULAR PAIN
H
↓PAIN-TEMP
LIGHT TOUCH AND
PROPRIOCEPTION INTACT

*Figure 10-5*

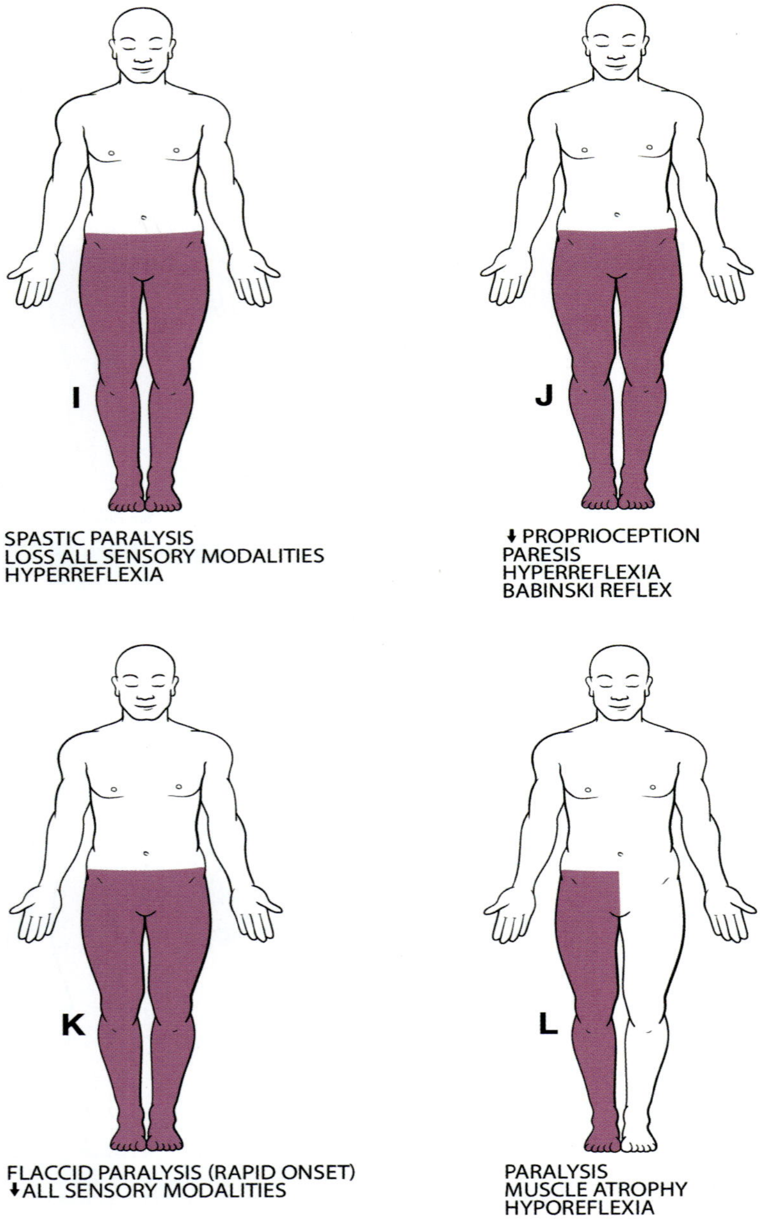
I
SPASTIC PARALYSIS
LOSS ALL SENSORY MODALITIES
HYPERREFLEXIA
J
↓ PROPRIOCEPTION
PARESIS
HYPERREFLEXIA
BABINSKI REFLEX
K
FLACCID PARALYSIS (RAPID ONSET)
↓ALL SENSORY MODALITIES
L
PARALYSIS
MUSCLE ATROPHY
HYPOREFLEXIA

*Figure 10-6*

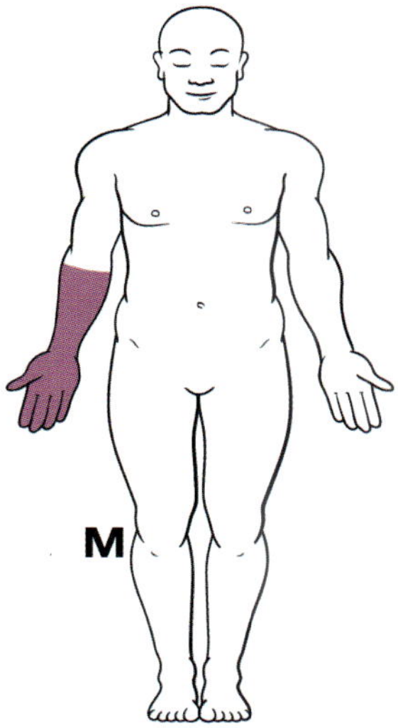


WEAKNESS - ELBOW AND
WRIST EXTENSION
NUMBNESS - DORSUM OF
HAND (RADIAL ASPECT)
↓TRICEPS REFLEX

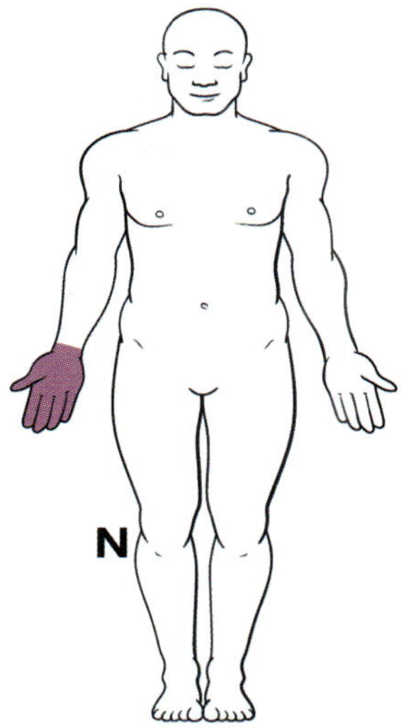


WEAKNESS - FLEXION OF WRIST,
THUMB, INDEX, AND MIDDLE FINGER
WEAKNESS - THUMB OPPOSITION
ATROPHY OF THENAR EMINENCE
PAIN - ALONG ABOVE FINGERS

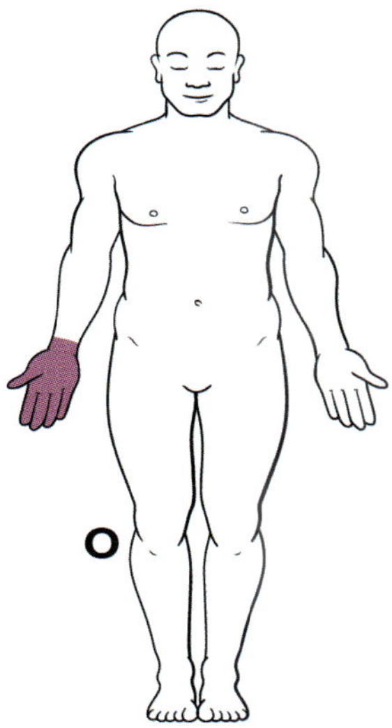


CLAW HAND
NUMBNESS - SMALL FINGER AND
ULNAR ASPECT OF THE RING FINGER
ATROPHY - HYPOTHENAR EMINENCE

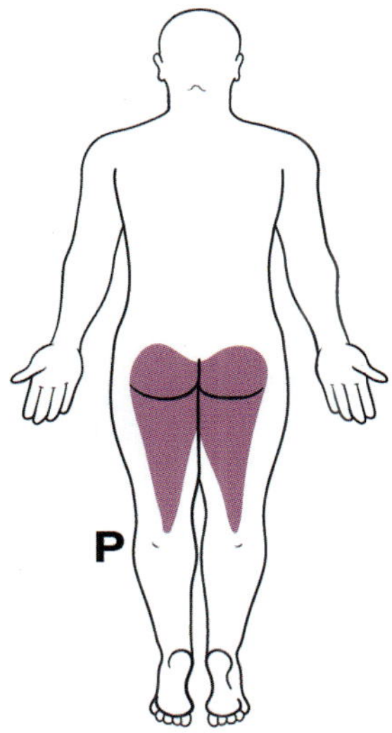


↓ALL SENSORY MODALITIES
ATROPHY
IMPOTENCE

*Figure 10-7*

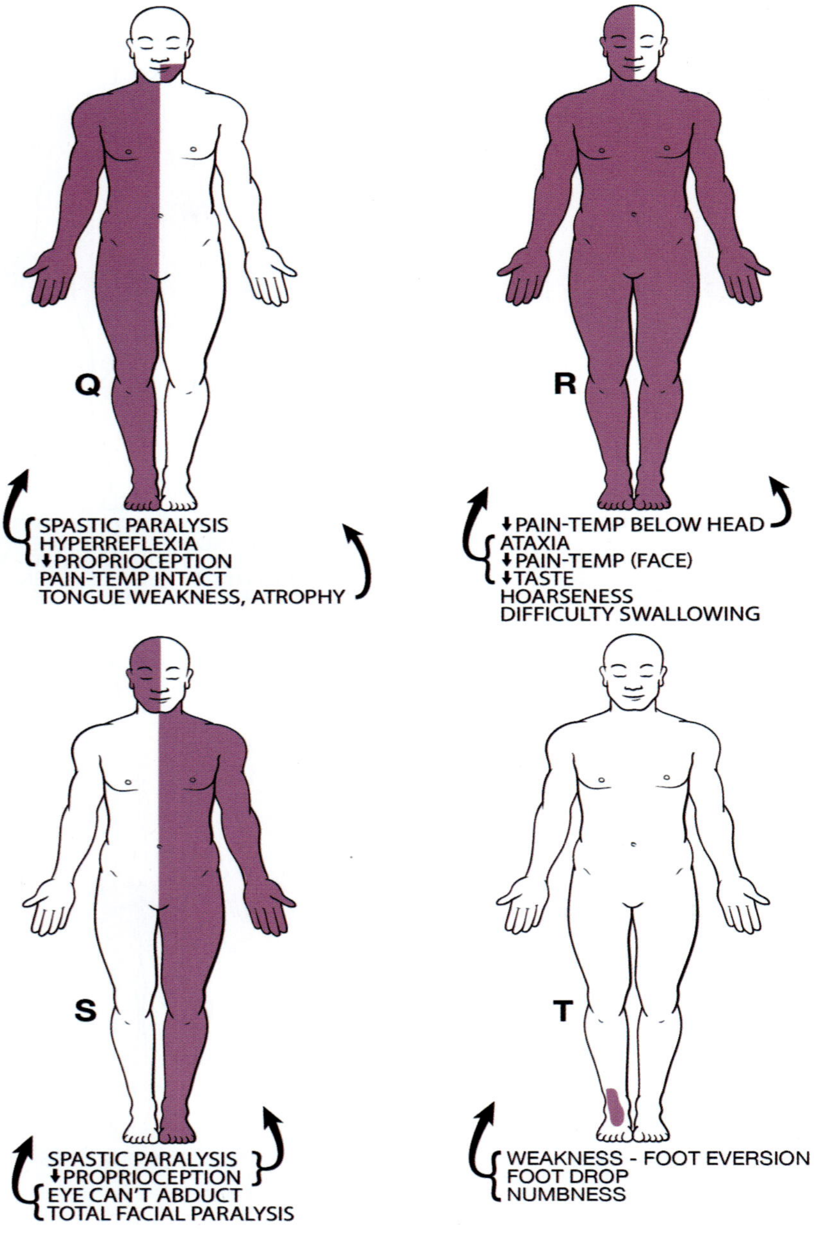
Q
SPASTIC PARALYSIS
HYPERREFLEXIA
↓PROPRIOCEPTION
PAIN-TEMP INTACT
TONGUE WEAKNESS, ATROPHY
R
↓PAIN-TEMP BELOW HEAD
ATAXIA
↓PAIN-TEMP (FACE)
↓TASTE
HOARSENESS
DIFFICULTY SWALLOWING
S
SPASTIC PARALYSIS
↓PROPRIOCEPTION
EYE CAN'T ABDUCT
TOTAL FACIAL PARALYSIS
T
WEAKNESS - FOOT EVERSION
FOOT DROP
NUMBNESS

*Figure 10-8*

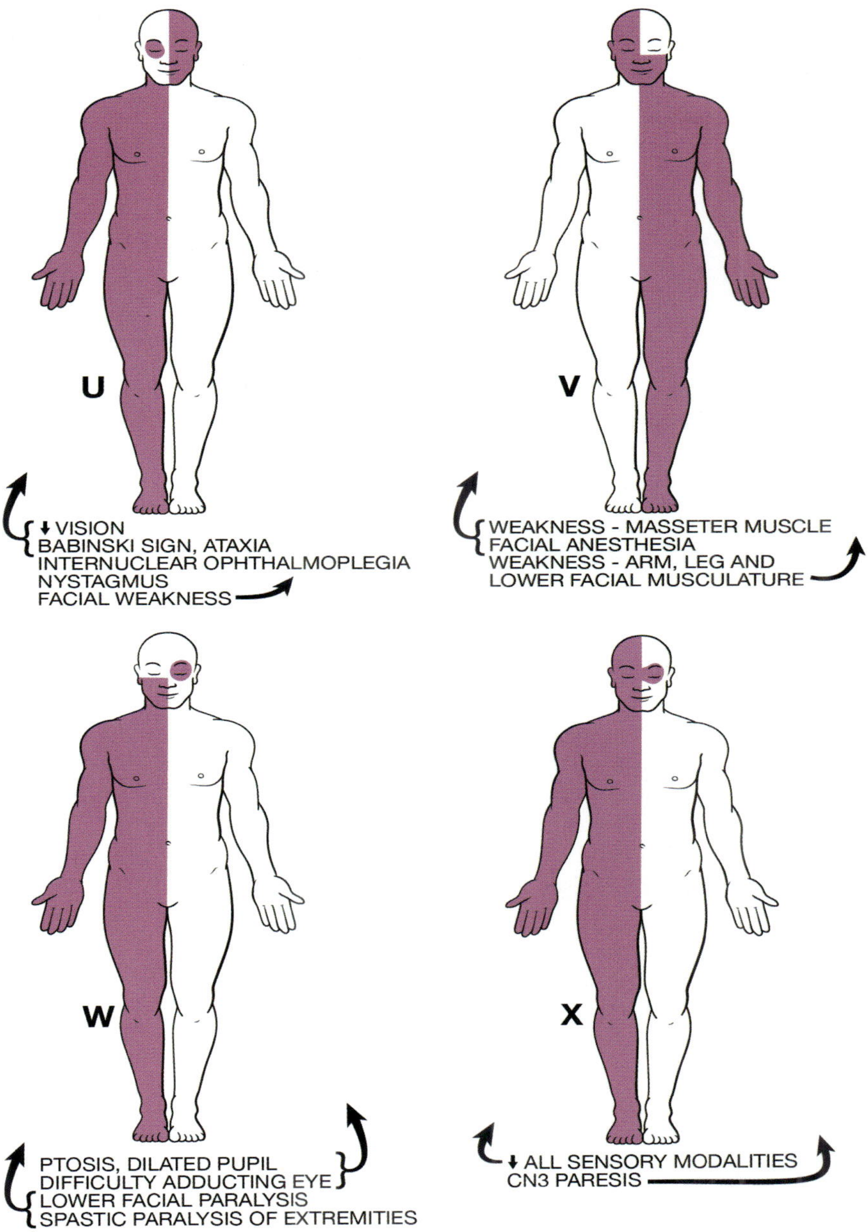
U
↓ VISION
BABINSKI SIGN, ATAXIA
INTERNUCLEAR OPHTHALMOPLEGIA
NYSTAGMUS
FACIAL WEAKNESS
V
WEAKNESS - MASSETER MUSCLE
FACIAL ANESTHESIA
WEAKNESS - ARM, LEG AND
LOWER FACIAL MUSCULATURE
W
PTOSIS, DILATED PUPIL
DIFFICULTY ADDUCTING EYE
LOWER FACIAL PARALYSIS
SPASTIC PARALYSIS OF EXTREMITIES
X
↓ ALL SENSORY MODALITIES
CN3 PARESIS

*Figure 10-9*

Answers to **Figs. 10-4** thru **10-9:**

A. Right anterior cerebral artery (supplies leg area of right cerebrum)(see **Figs. 2-2, 2-3**)
B. Right middle cerebral artery (see **Figs. 2-2, 2-3**)
C. Amyotrophic lateral sclerosis (Lou Gehrig's disease). Combination of upper and lower neuron signs (see **Fig. 3-5A**). Distal extremities commonly affected first.
D. Peripheral neuropathy (glove and stocking distribution)
E. Tertiary syphilis (tabes dorsalis). Upper extremities less commonly affected (see **Fig. 3-5B**)
F. Hemisection of spinal cord (Brown-Sequard syndrome) on left at T11. Loss of pain-temp on the right side with weakness and decreased proprioception on the left (see **Fig. 3-2**). (Pain-temp loss on the right side starts 1 or 2 vertebral segments below the lesion since crossing of the spinothalamic tract does not occur for 1 or 2 segments.
G. Radicular pain, cervical roots C5-C6
H. Syringomyelia C5-T2 (see **Fig. 3-5F**). Cervical levels are most affected, often with atrophy of the small muscles of the hand.
I. Total transection of spinal cord, T11. The deficit could also result from a midline tumor at the level of the central sulcus that affects both sides of the brain, but the deficit in the latter would probably be less dense than that following a spinal cord transection. In **transverse myelitis**, there is a cross-sectional lesion to one or more segments of the spinal cord due to an inflammation (transverse = cross-section; myelitis = spinal cord inflammation). The degree of deficit depends on the extent of inflammation, which may be due to an autoimmune disorder (e.g., multiple sclerosis, lupus), a viral or bacterial infection, or other inflammatory disorder.
J. Pernicious anemia. Commonly also presents with numbness and tingling of the distal portion of all extremities secondary to peripheral nerve involvement (see **Fig. 3-5C**)
K. Guillain-Barré syndrome. Commonly ascends to upper extremities and face after affecting lower extremities (see **Fig. 3-5E**)
L. Polio (see **Fig. 3-5D**)
M. Radial nerve injury
N. Median nerve compromise. When injury is at the level of the wrist (e.g., carpal tunnel syndrome), wrist flexion is unaffected.
O. Ulnar nerve injury
P. Cauda equina lesion, S2-S4
Q. Singe lesion to left medulla. Cranial nerve deficit (CN12) on left side (left tongue weakness and atrophy), corticospinal tract and medial lemniscus lesion on left side (spastic paralysis and decreased proprioception in right extremities)
R. Single lesion in right medulla (syndrome of the posterior inferior cerebellar artery). Lesion in right medulla to right CN5 sensory nucleus causes decreased pain-temp in right face; lesion to right spinocerebellar tract causes right-sided ataxia; lesion to right nucleus for taste (CN7) causes deficit for taste on right; lesion to right spinothalamic tract causes decreased pain-temperature in left extremities. Lesion to right vagus nerve nucleus causes hoarseness and difficulty swallowing. May also cause contralateral loss of facial pain-temp if right trigeminal lemniscus is involved (see **Fig. 4-3**)

S. Single lesion of the right caudal pons. Lesion to right CN6 (right eye can't abduct); lesion to right CN7 (total right face paralysis); lesion to right medial lemniscus (decreased proprioception left side of body); lesion to right corticospinal tract (spastic paralysis of left extremities)
T. Common peroneal nerve injury
U. Multiple sclerosis (no single lesion possible)
V. Single lesion to right pons. Lesion to right CN5 motor nucleus (right masseter weakness); lesion to right CN5 sensory nucleus (right facial anesthesia); lesion to right corticospinal tract (left-sided extremity weakness); lesion to right corticobulbar tract (left lower facial weakness)
W. Single lesion to left midbrain. Lesion to left CN3 (left ptosis, dilated left pupil, difficulty adducting left eye); lesion to left corticobulbar tract (CN7 right lower face weakness) and left corticospinal tract (right spastic paralysis of extremities
X. Single lesion to left midbrain. Lesion to left CN3 (left CN3 paresis); lesion to left medial lemniscus, left trigeminal lemniscus, and left spinothalamic tract (decrease in all sensation on the right)

# Part II. Neurologic History, Exam, and Treatment

# 11

# The Neurologic History

As in other areas of medicine, the history component of the neurologic examination frequently provides more useful information than the physical exam or laboratory tests. This section discusses key diagnostic questions in the evaluation of the most common symptoms and signs.

The neurologic history follows the same overall format as any general medical history. After eliciting the chief complaint, the history of the present illness must be taken carefully.

### *History of Present Illness*

Understand the main complaint:

a. What is the patient is feeling?
b. When did the problem begin and how did it progress? Problems arising acutely include vascular accidents; seizures; traumatic injury. Problems that evolve over time include degenerative brain disease, autoimmune, and inherited disorders. Some conditions have remissions and exacerbations, e.g., multiple sclerosis.
c. Is there anything that makes it feel better or worse? E.g., pressing on the site of a sinus or temporal arteritis headache is painful. In some people, pressing on the affected area of a cluster headache may make it feel better.
d. Are there any other associated symptoms? This information can give important clues as to a specific syndrome.

## Headache

*What type of pain is the patient feeling? Is it constant or throbbing*? Throbbing is more suggestive of a vascular cause. Intermittent lightning-like jabs over the trigeminal nerve distribution are characteristic of trigeminal neuralgia. Where is the headache located? Migraine headaches commonly show a predilection for one side of the head but should occur on the opposite side at least occasionally. If a headache always occurs only on the same side, suspect an underlying lesion, which will constantly refer pain to the same side of the head. Sinus headaches refer to the respective sinuses and are painful on direct pressure. The headaches of acute angle closure glaucoma and uveitis center around the eye and are associated with a red eye and visual loss. Tension headaches commonly refer to the top of the head, the neck, or to a band-like area around the temples and may include the eyes. The headache in meningitis and subarachnoid hemorrhage is likely to localize to the back of the neck; it is associated with neck stiffness during neck flexion, and often with pain spreading down the back due to inflammatory or red blood cells spreading down the cerebrospinal fluid.

*How did the headache progress?* A headache that has been intermittent over many years is less ominous than one that just recently occurred (particularly in an elderly person). The headache of subarachnoid hemorrhage characteristically occurs suddenly, whereas those of tumors generally progress over weeks or months.

*Does anything make the headache feel better or worse? How does it feel to press on the site of pain?* Infections or inflammations (as in sinusitis or temporal arteritis) usually feel worse on direct pressure. Tension and migraine headaches usually do not feel worse on direct pressure and often may feel better. *Is it worse in the day or at night*? Cluster headaches are severe unilateral headaches that occur particularly at night and often are worse with alcohol ingestion (they are also associated with a red eye). They commonly are "clustered," with remissions and exacerbations occurring over weeks or months. Headaches resulting from intracranial lesions may also occur at night. Trigeminal neuralgia attacks commonly are precipitated by chewing or touching a particular area of the face, such as the nose or mouth.

*Are there any other associated symptoms?* As the brain has no pain endings, commonly a tumor will first present with other neurologic findings (e.g., altered mental state, weakness, sensory loss, incoordination) before becoming large enough to affect pain endings in brain-contiguous structures, like the meninges. Suspect an extracranial source if pain is the only manifestation; most headaches have an extracranial origin.

*Do any other symptoms immediately precede the headache?* In classic migraine, there is a preceding aura, commonly a visual disturbance in one or both eyes (e.g., a wavy distortion, or scotoma, in front of one or both eyes, dizziness, nausea, and sometimes hemisensory or motor deficits).

## Dizziness

*What does the patient mean by "dizzy"?* Vertigo (a sense of spinning of the person or environment) suggests a lesion of the external vestibular apparatus, vestibular nerve, junction of vestibular nerve with the brain stem, or something occurring inside the CNS (central vertigo). "Lightheadedness" or "faintness" suggest impairment of brain oxygenation, as by cardiac arrhythmia, or hypotension, or psychological factors.

*Is the feeling worse on standing or lying down or during any particular activity?* Orthostatic hypotension improves on lying down. The vertigo of subclavian steal worsens on movement of the affected upper limb.

*Are there other associated symptoms?* Coinciding palpitations, angina, or shortness of breath should raise the question of a cardiac cause of dizziness.

## Visual Disturbance

*What is the patient experiencing?* Does the visual disturbance affect one or both eyes? Monocular visual loss indicates a problem anterior to the optic chiasm. Binocular problems originate at, or posterior to, the optic chiasm unless there are separate lesions of the optic nerves or retinae. **Figure 5-1** indicates the characteristic field defects in various conditions.

*Is the loss constant or intermittent?* Intermittent, brief visual loss is characteristic of transient ischemic attacks or migraine. In migraine the field often has a wavy appearance. In retinal detachment there is the feeling of a curtain being drawn over a particular sector of the eye, and it does not improve of its own accord. In acute (angle closure) glaucoma, the patient may see rainbows or halos on viewing lights. With digitalis toxicity the visual field may have a yellowish hue. With central scotomata, the patient has profound difficulty with reading, but otherwise can navigate fairly well because peripheral vision is intact. With peripheral field losses, the patient may read excellently but bumps into objects because side vision is defective.

*How did the problem begin and progress?* Acute visual loss suggests a vascular origin. Retinal detachment may progress over minutes or hours. Tumors may progress over months. Retinal degenerations may progress over years. Multiple sclerosis may be marked by remissions and exacerbations of visual loss over periods of weeks, months, or years.

*Does anything make the vision better or worse?* If the problem is improved by glasses or by reading at a particular distance, this indicates a refractive error.

*Are there other associated symptoms?* In migraine, the visual disturbance commonly precedes a throbbing headache and there may be other neurologic signs, like dizziness, nausea, weakness, or sensory loss. In uveitis and acute angle closure glaucoma, there may be intense pain about a red eye. In central nervous system lesions, there may be other neurologic signs suggesting the involvement of areas that border the visual pathways.

## Tremor

*Is it the fine tremor that often is seen with anxiety or in benign familial conditions? Or is it a coarse 4–6 cycle/second "pill-rolling" tremor that is commonly seen in Parkinson's disease?*

*Is the tremor worse when the limb is at rest or when doing something?* Parkinsonian tremor characteristically is worse at rest. Essential (benign, familial) tremor and tremors of cerebellar disease are worse on intention. Parkinsonian tremor (and that of anxiety) worsens on excitement and disappears during sleep.

*Are there any other associated symptoms?* In Parkinson's disease, stiffness and slowness of movements frequently accompany the tremor.

## Weakness And Sensory Loss

*Does the patient mean muscle weakness or is it a mental sense of "tiredness"? Is it "slowness", as in Parkinson's disease or myotonia?* In Parkinson's disease the strength may be normal, but the patient takes a long time to act. In myotonia, there may be slowness in release of a hand grasp. In myasthenia gravis, there may be initial good strength, developing into marked paresis on successive repetitions of the same act. *Does the patient who complains of "weakness" mean "pain" that decreases mobility, as in arthritis or bursitis?*

For sensory loss, when the patient says "numb," does this mean loss of feeling, or weakness? Patients sometimes use the term "numb" when describing weakness. *For "pain," "burning," "tingling," is it deep or superficial, the latter suggesting an involvement of cutaneous nerves as in herpes zoster, peripheral neuropathy, and other nerve dysfunctions.* Deep pain should call to mind additional potential factors –trauma, arthritis, inflammations, infections, or tumors.

*How did the weakness or sensory loss progress?* Strokes characteristically arise suddenly or are rapidly progressive over hours, then stabilizing. Transient ischemic attacks occur suddenly but then improve over a few minutes or hours. *Todd's paralysis* immediately following an epileptic seizure disappears within a few hours or days (there may also be transient sensory disturbances, visual defects, and aphasia). Tumors gradually progress and do not improve, with uncommon exceptions. Multiple sclerosis comes and goes intermittently over periods of weeks, months, or years. Symptoms of subdural hematomas may arise suddenly or progress over weeks if there is gradual expansion.

## Loss Of Consciousness

*In loss of consciousness, did the patient "fit and fall" or "fall and fit"?* That is, did a neurologic event precipitate the fall or did the fall occur accidentally, with the patient then hitting his head and losing consciousness? *Were there witnesses? Was there associated seizure activity, tongue biting, or urinary incontinence,* suggesting an epileptic seizure. Is there a prior history of a similar event? Is the patient taking any medication or have a cardiac history or mitigating event that may be implicated?

## Past History

Following the History of the Present Illness, a review of the patient's past general medical history may provide important information. A history of hypertension, diabetes, trauma, infection, tumors, allergies, surgery, cardiac, renal, hepatic, neurologic, or psychiatric illness may provide clues as to the origin of the neurologic symptoms.

The history of alcohol and other drug intake is particularly important as many drugs have neurologic side effects. The family-social history may reveal a relevant hereditary pattern, emotional stresses, or occupational exposure to toxic substances that relate to the problem.

A general physical exam may provide invaluable information, as neurologic symptoms often result from systemic diseases. Specific details of the neurologic component of the exam are presented in the following chapter.

# 12

# The Neurologic Exam

"NEURO WNL" ("The neurological exam is within normal limits") is commonly the last notation on a physical exam report. Regretfully, this often means that virtually no neuro exam took place. The patient kind of looked OK at a glance and had no particular neurologic complaints. A physician can be trapped into this approach, when there is inadequate time for the 90-minute neurologic exam some references suggest, or even the 20-minute exam suggested for patients with no neurologic complaints. There is, however, a brief neurologic screening exam that maximizes the useful information obtainable when time is limited. It is not a substitute for the more formal detailed evaluation that should follow when the screening exam reveals significant findings. This chapter describes this brief, but quickly informative, neurologic exam.

Mental status
Cranial nerves
Motor
Sensory
Coordination
Reflexes

## Mental Status

Key point: "FOGS"

1. **F**amily report of memory loss
2. **O**rientation
3. **G**eneral information
4. **S**pelling

In testing mental status during a neurological exam, a critical function one wishes to assess is memory, particularly recent memory. Recent memory tends to disappear before older memories when there is brain damage. Loss of recent memory functioning is the hallmark of the "organic brain syndrome" (*neurocognitive disorder*) that occurs with depressed brain function.

A useful term to remember is "FOGS" (as if one were testing how "foggy" one's mental state is):

First note how "foggy" the patient appears. Is the patient attentive? Or is there lethargy (tendency to drift off from attentiveness unless aroused), semicoma (arousal to noxious stimuli but not of sufficient degree to answer questions), or coma (lack of response to noxious stimuli). Rather than remember these definitions, it can help to simply describe what you notice. Then, if the patient is able, examine the individual components of the word "FOGS":

- **F - Family report**. Information, from a family member, that the patient has lost memory function is often a rapid and sensitive index of memory difficulty. A patient with a previously very high I.Q. may have dropped to a more average level not detectable on objective examination but identifiable on history. A history of memory decline obtained from a family member often will be more useful than a history of such obtained from the patient. The predominantly depressed patient, for instance, may exaggerate a problem of memory loss. The patient with a true dementia, on the other hand, may deny that there is a problem. If, however, the family reports that the patient is acting confused or is forgetful of things of late, this should raise the suspicion that at least a subtle form of cognitive decline exists, even if objective testing is normal.
- **O - Orientation**. Orientation as to precise time (month, day, year). Explain to the patient that you are asking routine questions and are interested in seeing how fast the patient responds. In this way you avoid insulting the patient with an elementary question. Orientation is useful, in that sometimes the patient appears normal superficially but will make the grossest error on this aspect of the exam (for instance, saying it is winter when it is summer, or that the year is 1935). Disorientation in identifying oneself, in the presence of preserved orientation for time and place, indicates a psychiatric disturbance.
- **G - General information**. "Who are the president and vice president of the United States?", or "What are some current events?" An "I don't know" may not be significant, as many people are ignorant of the news. An answer of "Roosevelt," however, establishes a gross dysfunction.

- **S - Spelling.** Ask the patient to spell the word "WORLD" forwards and backwards. Spelling "WORLD" forwards establishes that the patient can spell. If so, the patient should then be able to spell "WORLD" backwards. If not, this is a sign of neurocognitive disorder, the degree of which can be further quantitated by trying a four or three-letter word (e.g., "HAND," "CAT").

If the patient cannot spell, try numbers, as many people who are normally illiterate are still proficient in the use of numbers. For example:

a. Ask the patient to count backwards from 100 by 3's.
b. Ask the patient to repeat a 7-digit number. Most patients should be able to do this.

Alternatively, ask the patient to recall three objects (e.g., pencil, tie, table) several minutes after the examiner mentions them. The above questions, in a sense, are tests of short-term memory functioning. Spelling and calculation assess extremely short-term memory: i.e., the ability to concentrate and focus on the immediate task at hand.

## Cranial Nerves

**Cranial Nerve 1 (Olfactory Nerve)**
Key point: test each side with a mild agent (e.g., soap or coffee).

Testing the sense of smell seldom confirms significant pathology of the central nervous system. In fact, an abnormal finding may be confusing, as it may simply result from an obstructed nasal passage or be a normal decline in smell that occurs with aging (or COVID). It may be helpful, though, to test olfaction if there is suspicion of a frontal lobe lesion (for instance, change in personality; hemiparesis) or unexplained visual loss, as the olfactory pathways run under the frontal lobe near the optic chiasm.

Soap or coffee are usually readily available for testing olfaction. Ammonia should not be used as it stimulates the intranasal pain endings of the trigeminal nerve (CN5) rather than the olfactory nerve. The nasal septum divides the nasal passages into two, and olfaction should be tested on one side at a time.

**Cranial Nerve 2 (Optic Nerve)**
Key points:

1. Test visual acuity (near or far).
2. Test gross visual fields (finger confrontation).
3. Ophthalmoscopic exam

There are two particularly important aspects of vision to test:

A. *Central vision*, as tested by the Snellen chart (far vision) and / or the Rosenbaum pocket card (near vision). A nurse or other office aide can do this.
B. *Peripheral vision*, using gross visual fields.

**Central Vision**. The fovea, which lies in the center of the retina, is responsible for the sharp visual acuity of central vision. If the fovea is damaged, the patient will still be able to get around with peripheral vision but will have great difficulty reading. The patient with such a **central scotoma** usually comes to the doctor's office immediately, as lack of reading skill is a very noticeable deficit. Some patients, however, may not have noticed loss of vision in only one eye, as they never close one eye only. Thus, it is important to test for visual acuity in one eye at a time, even if the patient does not complain of visual loss. Usually, either the Snellen letter "far" chart or Rosenbaum "near" chart suffices. For illiterate patients an "E" chart or picture chart will suffice. The patient should wear her far glasses for far, and near glasses (or look through their bifocals) for near.

If you are not searching for a refractive problem but are only interested in determining whether a neurologic lesion is present in the visual pathway, then it suffices to test for either near or far vision. Bear in mind, however, that if one only uses the Rosenbaum near card,

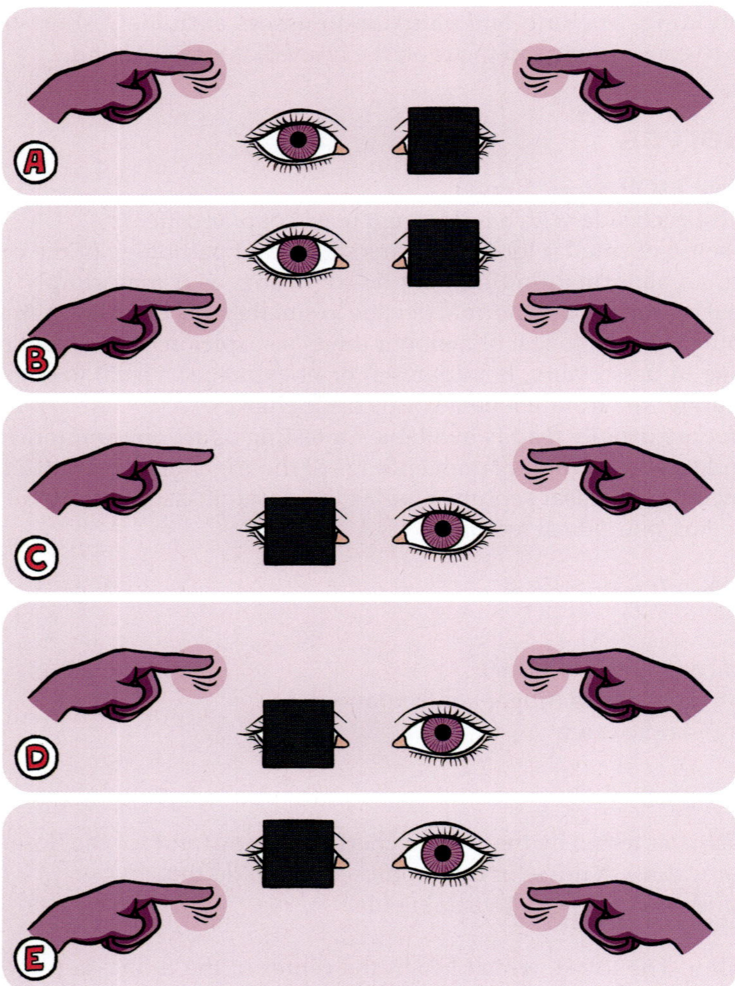


***Figure 12-1*** *Testing peripheral vision.*

one will not detect the nearsighted individual who has difficulty with far vision. Moreover, using the Snellen chart alone will not detect the farsighted or presbyopic individual who has headaches, blurry vision, and fatigue on near work. There is an additional advantage to testing both near and far vision: this can frequently distinguish visual loss that is due to a refractive error from that of a lesion (such as a cataract, or retinal or optic nerve damage). I.e., if the patient has good vision for far and poor vision for near (or vice versa) this implies a refractive error, which will be corrected by a change of glasses. If vision is poor and there is no difference between far and near vision, one must search more carefully for a lesion. The situation is analogous to a camera that gives blurry pictures. If the picture is clear at one distance but not another, there is a focusing (refractive) problem. If pictures are blurry at all distances, there could be an extreme focusing problem, but the origin may well be damaged film (retina) or a cloudy lens (cataract).

**Peripheral vision.** As for central vision, test one eye at a time. Otherwise, you may miss significant pathology that affects one eye only. **Figure 12-1** demonstrates a rapid visual field exam by gross confrontation, using finger motion, as follows:

A. Ask the patient to cover one eye and to look at your nose. Wiggle, simultaneously, the index fingers of your right and left hands in the superior fields. Ask the patient to point to, or state, the side that moved (the correct response is "both sides").
B. Repeat the same for the lower field.
C. Ask the patient now to cover the other eye. With both of your hands in the superior field, wiggle only your right index finger. The reason to not wiggle both fingers is that some patients, based on their experience with the first eye, may assume that the examiner is now going to always wiggle both fingers at once. Ask the patient to point to, or state, the side that moved.
D. Wiggle both fingers in the superior field. Ask where the motion is.
E. Wiggle both fingers in the inferior field. Ask where the motion is.

You have now generally tested peripheral vision. The Snellen and / or Rosenbaum charts tested central vision.

If there is the suspicion of a field defect, more subtle testing may be done by the neurologist or ophthalmologist, using a perimeter. Your gross motion testing has the advantage of rapidity, not requiring equipment, and is useful for the patient who has difficulty in maintaining a steady central focus.

Another important part of visual testing is the ophthalmoscopic examination. This can be performed either during the general physical exam or the neurologic exam. The ophthalmoscope can often detect the cause of visual loss:

a. The degree of severity of a cataract can be ascertained by the ease with which the fundus can be visualized. Generally, for cataracts, "If the examiner can see in, the patient can see out." Without the ophthalmoscope, the normal pupil looks *black*; with a dense cataract, it looks *white*. When looking through the ophthalmoscope, the normal pupil looks *red* due to the retinal red reflex; it looks *black* with a cataract, which blocks the red reflex.
b. Vitreous hemorrhages, retinal diseases, and optic atrophy can be detected as well as other conditions that relate to the neurologic status, such as papilledema (vision is typically normal initially in papilledema), and diabetic and hypertensive vascular

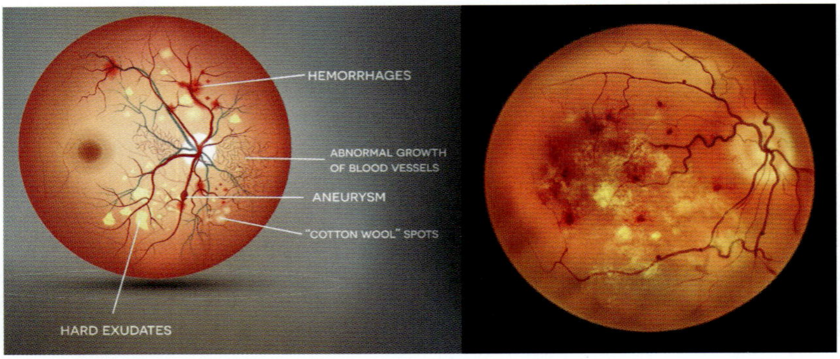


***Figure 12-2*** *Diabetic retinopathy.*

disease (**Figs. 11-2** and **11-3**)) (discussed in further detail in *Ophthalmology Made Ridiculously Simple,* by S. Goldberg and W. Trattler, Medmaster).

As a medical student, I once had an instructor who said that if you knew how to examine a retina, you know all of medicine. Years later, I came to realize that he was wrong – you can't know all of medicine by looking at a retina. The retina, though, does provide one place in the body where you can directly observe the state of blood vessels and nerve fibers.

Visual Field Loss Referrals :

- One eye blind = Think eye problem or optic nerve: Ophthalmology referral
- Same side visual field missing in both eyes = Think brain problem (e.g, stroke): Stroke workup
- Outer edge fields missing in both eyes = Think pituitary tumor: Urgent neurology + endocrine
- General rule: If a vision field problem affects both eyes the same way = Think brain problem

**Cranial Nerves 3, 4, 6**

Key tests:

1. Pupillary reaction to light
2. Lateral and vertical gaze

The term "PERLA" (pupils equal and responsive to light and accommodation) frequently appears on the physical exam report. Although this should mean that the examiner tested the normal pupillary constriction to light and to near accommodation, the accommodation part probably is rarely done routinely – nor is it likely to provide important information. True, a classic finding in tertiary syphilis is that the pupil (an irregular, small pupil) constricts on accommodation, which is normal, but not in response to light. However, tertiary syphilis is rare, and it is certainly unimportant to test the accommodation reaction if the response to light has already been found intact, which is the usual case. It suffices then, to test the response of each pupil to light and move on if that is normal (i.e., PERL).

Pupillary size sometimes is helpful to observe. A 20% difference in diameter between the right and left pupils is generally within the normal range of variability. A large, dilated

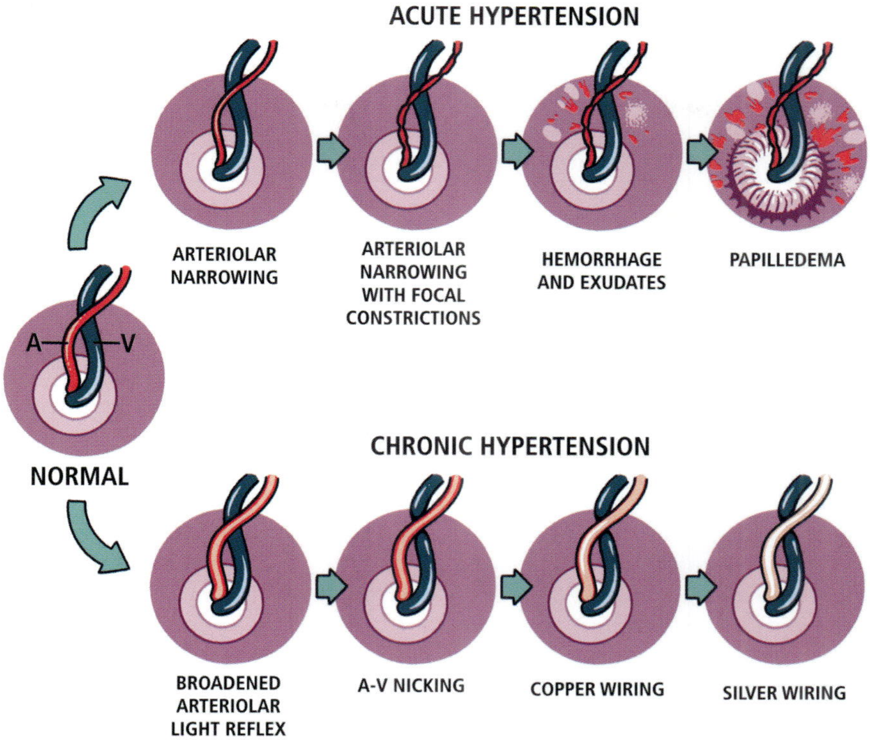


***Figure 12-3*** *Hypertensive retinopathy. (From Goldberg, S. and Trattler, W.* Ophthalmology Made Ridiculously Simple, *Medmaster)*

pupil on one side with no other ocular abnormalities is likely to be a benign variant, **Adie's pupil** (unless someone put dilating drops in the eye and didn't tell anyone). In Adie's pupil, the pupil reacts only slowly and slightly to a bright light; there are no other associated deficits of CN3. So don't rush to call the neurosurgeon. However, if the dilated pupil is due to CN3 injury inside or outside the brain stem, it is likely that this will be accompanied by other prominent neurologic symptoms - like diplopia or an altered state of consciousness. Examining pupillary size is particularly important when there is a depressed state of consciousness. A unilaterally dilated pupil in this setting may be due to herniation of the temporal lobe (uncal herniation) against CN3 and the brain stem.

The pupils may be markedly constricted with pontine injuries (pinpoint pupils) and with certain systemically administered drugs (e.g., *morphine, meperidine*). The pupil may be dilated in anoxia, as well as with certain systemically administered drugs (e.g., *atropine, scopolamine*).

Testing the pupillary response to light may help to confirm a lesion of CN2 or CN3 (**Figs. 5-3** and **12-4**).

Normally, shining a light in one eye causes both pupils to constrict (the *consensual reflex*), since the firing of the optic nerve ends up stimulating both sides of the brain stem (**Fig. 5-3**). If there is injury to one optic nerve (e.g., optic neuritis), say the right optic nerve, shining a light in the left eye will still cause both pupils to constrict (the consensual reflex). However,

| FIGURE 12-4. PUPILLARY REACTION FOLLOWING OPTIC OR OCULOMOTOR NERVE INJURY | | |
|---|---|---|
| **Injury** | **Light shine in right eye** | **Light shined in left eye** |
| Right optic nerve (CN2) | No response in either eye | Both pupils constrict |
| Right oculomotor nerve (CN3) | Only left pupil constricts | Only left pupil constricts |

rapidly moving the flashlight over the right eye will paradoxically cause the right pupil to *dilate* since it won't react to light, but only recover from the constriction caused by shining the light in the left eye.

Lateral and Vertical Gaze. Ask the patient to follow your finger, which you hold vertically and move horizontally back and forth, and then hold horizontally and move vertically back and forth. Ask how many fingers the patient sees (checking for diplopia). Also look for nystagmus.

If the patient reports diplopia with a particular finger position, note the position, as it will be useful in determining which eye muscle is involved, and then test one eye at a time; true diplopia should disappear when one eye is occluded, unless there is the rare occurrence of a dislocated lens, detached retina, or an irregularity in the corneal shape. (Note: Sometimes a patient says "double vision" but means blurry vision.)

Slight nystagmus at extreme lateral positions of gaze is normal. (Confirm this on a normal individual.) Marked nystagmus on extreme lateral gaze, or any nystagmus on forward gaze is abnormal. Jerk nystagmus, with a fast and slow component, suggests a peripheral or central nervous system lesion. Vertical nystagmus suggests a brain stem lesion. Pendular nystagmus (equal to-and-fro excursions) suggests a congenital condition, or blindness since early childhood. Ask the patient with pendular nystagmus whether the condition has always been present.

Pupil problems:

- One big pupil + confusion/headache = BRAIN HERNIATION: EMERGENCY - Get neurosurgery NOW
- One big pupil + no other symptoms = Probably benign: Ophthalmology referral
- Both small pupils = Drugs (opiates) or brain stem problem: Check drug screen, neurology if negative
- Both big pupils = Drugs (cocaine, amphetamines) or severe brain injury: Check drug screen, emergency if altered mental status
- Pearl: One big pupil + sick patient = EMERGENCY

Double vision problems:
Step 1: Cover one eye - does it go away?

- No = Not real double vision (blurry vision, eye problem)
- Yes = Real double vision, proceed to step 2

Step 2: Any other symptoms?

- Weakness, numbness, confusion = STROKE: Call stroke team
- Severe headache = Aneurysm: Emergency
- Just double vision = Cranial nerve problem: Neurology referral

Bottom line: Real double vision always needs neurology evaluation

Step 3: How fast did it start?
- Sudden = More urgent
- Gradual = Less urgent but still needs workup

**Cranial Nerve 5 (Trigeminal nerve)**

Key test: *Double simultaneous stimulation*, with pin (or toothpick acting as a pin, to avoid patient contamination from a repeatedly used pin) or light touch. Double simultaneous stimulation is done as follows: Touch both sides of the face simultaneously. Ask what the patient feels. If the patient consistently reports sharpness (or light touch) on one side only, this suggests a significant sensory defect on the dull side. If both sides are reported sharp with the toothpicks, a more sensitive assessment can be made by keeping the toothpicks in place and repeating the question 5 or 10 seconds later. If the patient now reports that only one side is sharp (**extinction**), this points to a subtle sensory deficit on the dull side. This *sensory adaptation* is a more subtle way of assessing pain deficit than testing each side of the cheek separately.

A CNS lesion that compromises CN5 sensory function most likely will involve all three divisions of CN5, so it is really only necessary to test one point on each cheek on routine exam, to rule out CNS compromise of CN5. If a peripheral nerve lesion of CN5 causes a sensory deficit over one of the three CN5 dermatomes (ophthalmic, maxillary, mandibular), most likely the patient will report this without your having to perform an exam. Thus, testing all three divisions is generally unnecessary unless the patient reports a sensory loss over a particular nerve division or there is some other reason to suspect a nerve division lesion. It is also unnecessary to test the corneal blink reflex (on touching the cornea with a wisp of cotton) unless one already suspects a CN5 or CN7 lesion. The corneal blink reflex depends on CN5 to relay sensation to the brain stem and on CN7 (facial nerve) to cause constriction (bilaterally) of the orbicularis oculi muscles (CN7). This test is useful to confirm a deficit of either CN5 or CN7 in the eye region.

**Cranial Nerve 7 (Facial nerve)**

Key test: Smile.

Testing this nerve is a critical part of the neurologic examination. Ask the patient to smile, noting whether there is weakness, on either side, of elevation of the corner of the mouth. Often, weakness is apparent even without this maneuver, as there is noticeable flattening of the nasolabial fold. Lesions of the cerebral cortex or its pathway to the motor nucleus of the facial nerve in the pons will cause contralateral weakness of the mouth - but not the forehead. Thus, the typical cerebral stroke results in weakness in elevating the corner of the mouth but no significant weakness in wrinkling the brow (**Fig. 4-4**). In Bell's palsy, or other forms of peripheral nerve damage to CN7, where the nerve is injured between the pons and face, there is total facial paralysis on one side: i.e., weakness of elevating the corner of the mouth as well as closing the eye and wrinkling the brow. Thus, if there is weakness of the mouth, one must test for weakness of brow wrinkling to determine whether the lesion is central or peripheral. On the other hand, if elevation of the corner of the mouth is normal (as is true in the great majority of physical examinations), there is little point in continuing further the examination of CN7, as one is not likely to find a paralysis of the brow and eyelid without a weakness of the lower face.

In summary, is the facial droop stroke or Bell's palsy?:

STROKE (Upper Motor Neuron):

- Forehead wrinkles NORMALLY (can raise eyebrow)
- Lower face weak
- Other stroke signs (arm/leg weakness, speech problems)
- GET STROKE TEAM

Bell's Palsy (Lower Motor Neuron):

- Whole face weak (can't close eye, can't raise eyebrow)
- No other symptoms
- Starts over hours-days (not sudden)
- Neurology referral (not emergency)

Even more briefly: If forehead works = brain problem (stroke)
If forehead doesn't work = nerve problem (Bell's palsy)

**Cranial Nerve 8 (Vestibulocochlear nerve)**

Key test: Hear fingertips moving near the ear

With your fingers near the ears of the patient, rub together the thumb and index fingers of either your right or left hand. Ask the patient to point to the ear in which the patient hears the sound. This is a rapid screen for hearing. If there is a defect, determine whether it is a conductive defect (e.g., wax in the ear, damaged ear drum or ossicles) or a sensorineural defect. This can be accomplished without tuning forks simply by asking the patient to hum. In conductive defects (defect in the outer or middle ear), the poorly hearing ear hears the hum louder. In sensorineural deficits (damage to the cochlea or auditory nerve), the normal ear hears the hum louder. (Try this by sticking a finger in your ear and humming. The ear with the finger in it hears the sound louder.)

**Cranial Nerves 9, 10 (Glossopharyngeal, Vagus)**

Key test: Gag reflex.

These nerves are tested together by inducing a brief gag reflex. This may be performed when one examines the pharynx and depresses the tongue with a tongue depressor. Touch the soft palate or pharynx. When the gag occurs, note whether the soft palate retracts symmetrically. If the nerve injury is one-sided, the palate will retract to the normal side. Compromise of these nerves is extraordinarily rare, and generally this unpleasant test can be omitted.

**Cranial Nerve 11 (Accessory nerve)**

Key test: Shoulder elevation.

This nerve is rarely damaged except during neck injuries. This simple test generally suffices: Ask the patient to raise their shoulders (trapezius contraction) against the manual resistance of the examiner. One can also test for sternocleidomastoid function by assessing the strength of lateral head rotation against the manual resistance of the examiner, but this is generally unnecessary, unless the result of trapezius testing is abnormal.

**Cranial Nerve 12 (Hypoglossal nerve)**

Key test: Stick out the tongue.

If there is weakness on one side of the tongue, the tongue will deviate to that side. It is rare for this nerve to be affected, but the test is easy to perform. (Mnemonic: Imagine you're pushing the handlebars of a bicycle. If your left hand becomes weak, the wheel will turn to the left. Similarly, when your left tongue is weak, the tongue will deviate to the left on protrusion.)

Cranial Nerve Red Flags:

CN2 (Vision): Sudden vision loss = Emergency (stroke, GCA)

CN3 (Eye movement): Dilated pupil + eye doesn't move = Emergency (herniation)

CN5 (Face sensation): Numb face = Usually not emergency

CN6 (Eye movement): Double vision = Urgent neurology referral

CN7 (Face movement): Face droop = Stroke vs Bell's palsy (check forehead - weak in Bell's palsy)

CN8 (Hearing): Sudden deafness = Emergency (steroid window - better results if started early)

Simple Rule: Any SUDDEN cranial nerve problem = get help fast

## Extremities: Motor Exam

Key tests:

1. Drift of upper extremity (and of lower extremity if there is a question of lower extremity weakness)
2. Hand grasp and toe and foot dorsiflexion
3. Testing of other muscles, when their proper function is in question

If one had all the time in the world, one could try to test every joint in the body for flexion, extension and other movements. By understanding the major aims of the examination, the approach may be shortened. If the examiner wishes to determine whether there has been a lesion to the brain stem or cerebrum that has caused extremity weakness, one of the simplest, most rapid, and subtle tests is for drift: Ask the patient to close their eyes and hold their arms horizontally forward, palm up for about 15–30 seconds. If there is weakness of the upper extremity, the hand on the affected side will slowly drop or rotate inward (pronate). (While waiting to observe for drift, time may be saved by simultaneously testing something else, such as strength of toe and foot dorsiflexion.)

To test lower extremity drift, have the patient lie on their stomach, with knees bent and legs pointing vertically. Within about ½ minute, the leg on the weak side will tend to waver and drop. A common motor pattern in cerebral hemisphere stroke is drift and flattening of the nasolabial fold on the weak side. There may also be a homonymous hemianopia of the visual field on the weak side. Weakness of hand grasp and toe and foot dorsiflexion are also commonly seen in upper motor neuron injury. An easy, non-awkward way to test the strength of a hand grasp is for you to cross your hands and ask the patient to grasp your index and middle fingers (try it and you'll see why crossing your hands is less awkward). The patient will grasp your right fingers with his right hand and left fingers with his left hand. Determine the ease with which you can pull your fingers out. Toe and foot dorsiflexion are tested by asking the patient to move the toe and foot against the manual resistance of the examiner.

If you suspect a peripheral injury to nerve or muscle (e.g., the patient presents with local numbness along a dermatome, pain radiating down the extremity, a history of trauma to the neck or extremity, or complaints of weakness of an extremity of uncertain cause), then more formal testing of the extremity is in order. It is simplest to remember to test all the joints for all their kinds of motion. I.e., test flexion and extension of the shoulder, elbow, wrist, and fingers; abduction of the shoulder and fingers; opposition of the thumb and small finger, etc. Opposition may be tested by having the patient hold a piece of paper tightly between the thumb and another finger, while the examiner attempts to pull away the paper.

The motor exam will be invalid if the patient cannot perform because of pain.

In Parkinson's disease, a stepwise "cogwheel" rigidity may be felt on passive flexion and extension of the joints, particularly the wrist.

## Extremities: Sensory Exam

Key tests:

1. Pain sensation–use double simultaneous stimulation
2. Proprioception–test big toe

### *Pain*

It is rarely useful to test all the dermatomes and turn the patient into a pincushion. Generally, if a patient has loss of sensation, or tingling, or burning over a particular dermatome, they will outline the strip-like dermatome area with their own fingers. This will obviate the need for extensive pin testing, except for confirmation in the region outlined by the patient. Cerebral lesions (e.g., stroke, tumor) do not present as dermatome deficits; with cerebral lesions there is more likely to be a general area deficit, such as the whole extremity. When testing for pain sensation in a suspected cerebral lesion, **double simultaneous stimulation** is a very subtle and rapid test, as follows:

Take two toothpicks (less germy than reused safety pins) and position them on the dorsum of the patient's hands (their hands are resting on their lap with eyes closed). Ask the patient what they feel on each hand – "sharp" or "dull" (this may require a previous demonstration to the patient as to what is meant by sharp and dull). Bilaterally apply the toothpicks. If the patient consistently reports sharpness on one side only, this suggests a significant sensory deficit on the dull side. If both hands are reported sharp, keep the toothpicks in place and repeat the question 5 or 10 seconds later. If the patient now consistently reports that only one side is sharp (**extinction**), this points to a subtle deficit on the dull side. This sensory adaptation is a key to the double simultaneous stimulation test and is a more rapid and subtle way of assessing pain deficit than is testing each hand separately.

Perform a similar maneuver for the cheeks (testing CN5, if not already done) and the dorsum of the feet.

## *Proprioception—Stereognosis*

Key test: Proprioception of big toe.

Have the patient close their eyes. Bend the big toe into either a plantarflexed or dorsiflexed position. Ask the patient to state whether the toe is "down" or "up" (this may require a previous demonstration to the patient as to what is meant by down or up). Consistent errors suggest a proprioceptive problem. Be sure to grasp the toe at its sides, as grasping on the posterior and plantar surfaces may induce pressure that inadvertently gives the patient position clues.

Conditions that commonly cause proprioceptive difficulty (e.g., multiple sclerosis, neurosyphilis, pernicious anemia) are likely to affect the lower extremity before the upper extremity. Thus, it generally is unnecessary to test the upper extremities if the lower extremities are normal, unless there are other obvious problems with the upper extremity (e.g., trauma to the neck or upper extremity causing numbness or loss of motor function).

The testing of vibration (preferably with a low pitch C-128 tuning fork applied to the bony part of the wrist and ankle) provides another way of assessing posterior column pathway deficits. Using yourself as a control, ask the patient when the vibration disappears. Generally, though, proprioceptive testing suffices. Elderly people may normally have decreased vibratory sense; finding an absence of vibratory sense can lead to the mistaken impression of a significant neurologic deficit.

Testing for stereognosis (e.g., the ability to identify a coin by touch alone) generally is not crucial, since proprioception, vibration, and stereognosis information travels along the same pathways, the posterior columns of the spinal cord, and testing proprioception generally suffices. However, it is helpful to know that the peripheral receptors for proprioception and vibration differ and sometimes may be differentially affected in disease. Moreover, stereognosis has more complex circuitry in the brain to identify what one is feeling. So, there are occasions where it might be helpful to test all three senses. It is generally unnecessary to test temperature if pain sensation is normal, but if there is a question, temperature can be tested using a container filled with warm water and a cool object like the tuning fork.

## *Light touch*

Double simultaneous stimulation (by grazing the skin or hair lightly with your hand or, more sensitively, with a wisp of cotton) provides a sensitive measure of light touch.

# Coordination

Key tests:

1. Finger-to-nose and heel-to-shin
2. Rapid alternating movements of hand and foot.

The theoretical aim of this aspect of the exam is the testing of cerebellar and basal ganglia function, as these structures play such an important role in coordination. However, vision, proprioception and vestibular sense (and muscle strength) also play an important role in coordination and must be considered in making an assessment.

Basal ganglia lesions tend to be characterized by unintended movements while at rest (e.g., resting tremor, athetosis, chorea, hemiballismus). Hence, they are generally detectable simply by observing the resting patient. For instance, in Huntington's chorea, there may be inadvertent squirming movements of the extremities and head. In Parkinson's disease, the tremor is characteristically worse with the extremity at rest, improving with motion, as in reaching for an object.

Cerebellar lesions result in awkwardness of intended movements and are best analyzed by asking the patient to perform specific movements. For example:

- Finger-to-nose and heel-to-shin. Have the patient close their eyes, hold out their hands laterally, and then touch the tip of their nose. Successive repetitions of this movement will help to detect any awkwardness. In heel-to-shin testing, the patient slowly tries to move their heel along the front of the shin from the knee to ankle and back to the knee. Awkwardness of this action should raise the question of a cerebellar pathway lesion (assuming that conscious proprioception is intact and there is no major weakness).
- Rapid alternating movements. Have the patient repeatedly and rapidly tap their thumb and index finger against one another. Test right and left hands simultaneously. (Or have the patient place their hands, palms down, on their lap and alternately supinate and pronate rapidly.) For the lower extremity, have the patient place their heel on the floor and rapidly tap their foot. Test one foot at a time. Slowness may result from a cerebellar lesion, proprioceptive defect, or paresis.

If there is a problem with balance, **tandem gait** and the **Romberg test** should also be performed:

In tandem gait, the patient should be able to walk placing one foot successively in front of the other, i.e., walk heel-to-toe. The Romberg test is useful to distinguish among the causes of balance difficulty, as follows:

There are three senses which aid in maintaining one's balance: *vision, vestibular sense,* and *proprioception*. These senses feed directly or indirectly into the cerebellum. The patient must have two out of 3 of these senses intact to maintain balance. Thus, closing the eyes normally eliminates one sense, but the other two still function, and the patient will not sway. If proprioception is lacking, the patient will keep their balance with the eyes open but sway with the eyes closed.

If the latter occurs, the Romberg test is "positive." A positive Romberg implies a proprioceptive or vestibular malfunction. If the patient sways with or without the eyes open, consider a cerebellar lesion; it is as if none of the sensory inputs can filter through the cerebellum to achieve proper functioning. (The test in that case, semantically, is considered "negative"; the definition of "Romberg positive" is swaying when the eyes are closed, but no swaying when the eyes are open.) Suspicion of a vestibular deficit can be confirmed by the report of vertigo (sensation that the patient or environment is spinning). Suspicion of a proprioceptive deficit is confirmed by an abnormality in proprioceptive testing. Evidence of a visual deficit is confirmed, of course, by checking visual acuity.

Difficulty in balance may also occur with a blood pressure drop, especially in orthostatic hypotension. In this, the patient tends to complain of dizziness, or lightheadedness (as opposed to vertigo, a spinning sensation) in an upright position. Orthostatic hypotension is tested by checking the blood pressure in the supine and erect positions. Normally, there should not be a drop greater than 20 mm Hg of systolic pressure (or 10 mm Hg diastolic blood pressure) within 3 minutes of standing.

Balance difficulty may also occur with weakness or rigidity of the lower extremities.

## Reflexes

The major reflexes are the triceps, biceps, knee jerk, ankle jerk, and Babinski sign. A normal individual may have very active or absent reflexes bilaterally; asymmetry of the reflex responses is generally more significant for pathology. In using the reflex hammer, one will obtain a more reliable reflex if the hammer is held loosely and swung between the fingers, than if it is grasped firmly in the palm.

A positive **Babinski reflex** is an important sign that points to an upper motor neuron lesion. In this test, the lateral aspect of the foot is scratched slowly with a pointed object. Normally, the toes respond with plantar flexion. A positive Babinski sign is characterized by abnormal dorsiflexion of the big toe, accompanied by a fanning out of the toes. The test should not be performed in such a stimulating manner as to cause dorsiflexion of the ankle; an upgoing toe in that case could simply be due to ticklishness. An asymmetric response is particularly significant. Abdominal, cremasteric, and jaw jerk flexes generally are not necessary to test, as other aspects of the history and exam are likely to provide more valuable confirmative information.

The hyperreflexia of an upper motor neuron lesion, when pronounced, may be accompanied by **clonus**. Clonus is an involuntary rhythmic alternating jerking muscle contraction and relaxation that occurs in response to a sudden stretch of muscle, e.g., sudden dorsiflexion of the ankle by the examiner.

Tests for meningeal irritation:

The **Kernig** and **Brudzinski** signs are tests for meningeal irritation, as occurs in meningitis and subarachnoid hemorrhage. These tests should be performed in patients with unexplained posterior headaches, fever, or altered mental state. In the Brudzinski test the head is flexed by the examiner; the patient with meningeal irritation reports marked pain in the back of the neck and responds with flexion of the hip and lower extremities. In the Kernig test, the patient reports pain in the lower back when the examiner raises a straightened right or left lower extremity. Such pain on straight leg raising is also found unilaterally, however, with low back muscle spasm and sciatic nerve irritation, as may occur with a herniated disc.

The **Chvostek** and **Trousseau signs** can be detected in hypocalcemia. The Chvostek sign is elicited by tapping or lightly tapping the facial nerve in front of the earlobe. This causes twitching of the facial muscles. The Trousseau sign can be seen on inflating a blood pressure cuff on the upper arm above systolic blood pressure for a few minutes. This causes carpal spasm or flexion of the wrist (resembling a claw) in hypocalcemia.

## Evaluation Of The Unconscious Patient

Key points:

1. ABCs first: Airway, Breathing, Circulation. Get help if available.
2. Pupils. One big pupil = herniation emergency
3. Purposeful movement: Does the patient try to push you away?
4. Babinski reflex: Both up = severe brain injury
5. Abnormal eye movements
6. Hand drop from over head

Think causes:

- Drugs/alcohol: Most common (check pupils)
- Stroke: Sudden onset, focal signs
- Seizure: Usually wake up after (post-ictal)
- Infection: Fever, neck stiffness
- Check blood sugar (easiest fix)

Of course, it is necessary at the outset to establish that pulse and respiration are intact, as cardiopulmonary resuscitation may be required before proceeding with the neurologic exam. The history from accompanying relatives or friends also is very important, particularly regarding drug intake, trauma, seizure history, or metabolic, cardiac, or neurologic disease.

An important aim of the neurologic exam is to determine whether any asymmetries exist in neurologic function. If so, this shifts the likely diagnosis away from a metabolic cause and toward that of a structural lesion, as metabolic problems are more likely to affect the body symmetrically.

**Handrop**. To determine malingering or hysterical (conversion disorder) loss of consciousness, raise the patient's hand over his head and drop it. If it strikes his face, this suggests a physiologic problem. If it misses, this suggests a nonphysiologic cause, as a conscious patient tries to avoid striking himself. Alternatively, cold caloric testing can be used. A 20 cc syringe is filled with cold water and attached to a piece of IV tubing. The tube is inserted into the patient's ear (check first to rule out a perforated drum, as performance of the test may then be damaging). The water is introduced over a 5 to 10 second period. In normal patients, there is nystagmus with the slow component toward the water (**Fig. 5-6**). In coma, there is no nystagmus and there may be no response at all. In intermediate stages (stupor, obtundation), there will be net deviation of the eyes to the cold water, with or without nystagmus. In malingering or conversion disorder the response will be normal.

## Benji

One day, a neighbor frantically knocked on my door and told me that she could not arouse her 6-year-old son, Benji. I raced over to the house to find Benji lying on the couch, and indeed it did not seem possible to awaken him. A preliminary neurologic exam revealed nothing wrong. I then raised Benji's arm above his face and let go. Benji's hand fell to the side and missed his face.

I then announced to Benji, that since I could not wake him up, I would have to give him a big shot in the behind with a needle that he would not feel since he was not awake, and that I was going out of the room to prepare the shot. I left the room with Benji's parents and came back about a minute later. Benji was gone. He was hiding behind the couch.

So arriving at a complex diagnosis is not always difficult when there is a pearl that shows the way.

The number of neurologic functions that can be tested in a comatose patient is limited because of the lack of patient cooperation. The most important tests are:

**Pupillary size and response to light**. *Bilateral pinpoint pupils* suggest either a drug effect (e.g., morphine, meperidine, heroin, propoxyphene, methadone, barbiturates), or a structural lesion (e.g., pontine hemorrhage). *Bilateral large pupils* may occur with other drugs (e.g., atropine and other anticholinergics, sympathomimetics such as amphetamines or pseudoephedrine, cocaine, methylphenidate, LSD), with diffuse anoxia, or with structural lesions.

Asymmetric pupils (greater than 20% difference) should raise the suspicion of a structural lesion. If the asymmetry is that of an Adie's pupil (long history of the asymmetry and no other ocular signs except for a pupil that reacts very slowly to light), this is inconsequential. If it is due to CN3 compromise, this may be life-threatening, as there may be an uncal herniation against the brain stem and CN3. If the affected eye also has a ptosis and is down-and-out, this strongly points to a CN3 lesion.

A fixed dilated pupil on one side is a potentially grave sign in a comatose patient, and the neurosurgeon must be contacted immediately. There is high risk of brain herniation causing damage to CN3 and the brain stem.

The blink reflex that occurs with corneal stimulation tests both cranial nerves 5 and 7. Absence of the reflex suggests brain stem compromise or peripheral nerve injury to cranial nerve 5 or 7, although the reflex may be absent in severe metabolic encephalopathies.

**Abnormal eye movements.** A tendency for the eyes to deviate to one side should raise the suspicion of a cerebral or brain stem lesion. In cerebral lesions the eyes tend to "look toward the lesion," because each hemisphere controls eye movements to the opposite side. The direction of gaze may vary with brain stem lesions. Ocular divergence or roving eye movements, with the eyes moving in asymmetric ways, should raise the suspicion of brain stem depression.

The **Doll's Eye reflex** may be a useful test for brain stem injury. In this test, one turns the patient's head suddenly to one side and observes whether the eyes lag behind. This is similar to a doll's eye which maintains the same position when the head is tilted back. The response is absent in coma. The reflex is believed to be brain stem mediated, and a total lack of response is believed to reflect significant brain stem dysfunction. Of course, before performing this exam, it is wise to know that the patient does not have a broken neck.

**Response to noxious stimulus**. Twist your knuckle into the patient's sternum, thereby inducing a noxious stimulus. Unless the patient is in deep coma, the patient should attempt to resist by reflex bending of the leg or arm, or grimacing. If these responses are asymmetric, this suggests a structural lesion.

**The Babinski reflex**. An asymmetric Babinski reflex indicates an upper motor lesion. A bilateral Babinski reflex in most cases indicates bilateral involvement of the CNS. It is normal, though, in infants $< 2$ years of age.

In **locked-in syndrome**, commonly from a stroke or other brain injury that affects the pons, the patient is conscious but is paralyzed and cannot communicate, except for the ability to look up and blink. To determine this, ask the patient to look up or blink. Blinking may become an important mode of communication, not only in response to questions but with devices that can track eye movements and translate them into cursor movements on a computer screen.

**Super Brief Essential Exam**

MENTAL STATUS (2 minutes):
- Alert and oriented x 3 (person, place, time)
- Follow simple commands
- Remember 3 words after 5 minutes
- Red flag: Can't remember 3 words = cognitive problem

CRANIAL NERVES (3 minutes):
- Vision: Read something, check visual fields roughly
- Pupils: Equal, round, reactive to light
- Eye movements: Follow your finger, any double vision?
- Face: Smile (symmetric?), feel both sides of face
- Hearing: Whisper in each ear
- Swallow: Any trouble with voice/swallowing?

MOTOR (3 minutes):
- Strength: Test major muscle groups (5/5 scale)
- Tone: Floppy vs stiff vs normal
- Coordination: Finger to nose, heel to shin

SENSORY (2 minutes):
- Light touch: Both sides of arms/legs
- Vibration: Tuning fork on big toes
- Don't test everything - focus on patient's complaints

REFLEXES (2 minutes):
- Biceps, knees, ankles
- Babinski: Stroke bottom of foot (toe up = abnormal)

GAIT (1 minute):
- Walk normally, then heel-to-toe

# 13

# Neurologic Imaging

Gastroenterology has the luxury of directly visualizing and biopsying a lesion through endoscopy. Neurology does not. To view directly into the skull, brain stem, or spinal column, the neurologist must rely on imaging techniques, and these have become sophisticated.

## X-Rays

Plain X-rays of the skull and spine are useful in discovering bony defects, such as fractures or tumor erosion. Plain X-rays are severely limited in their ability to distinguish one area of soft tissue from another or to distinguish soft tissue from fluid compartments.

## Computerized Axial Tomography (CAT; CT) Scan

The CAT scan has revolutionized neurological diagnosis. This form of X-ray, which shows the brain as a series of sections, whether coronal or horizontal, can easily differentiate areas of the ventricular system from areas of soft tissue and can delineate individual neural structures and lesions from surrounding regions. The procedure is even more effective with intravenously injected iodinated contrast material, which enhances lesions of various kinds. Tumors, hemorrhages, vascular abnormalities, abscesses, and ventricular dilation, which cannot be seen on routine X-ray, can be seen on the CAT scan (**Figs. 13-1, 13-2, 13-3**). The CAT scan is particularly useful in distinguishing strokes due to infarction versus strokes that result from hemorrhage.

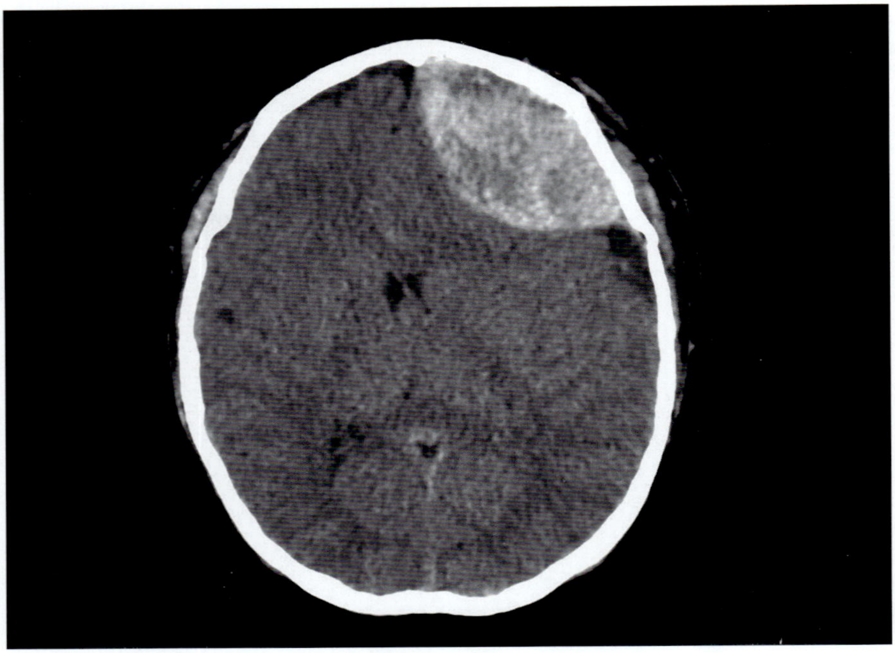

***Figure 13-1*** *CAT scan showing characteristic biconvex (lens-shaped) epidural hemorrhage. The shape is constrained by the firm dural attachments to the skull bone.*

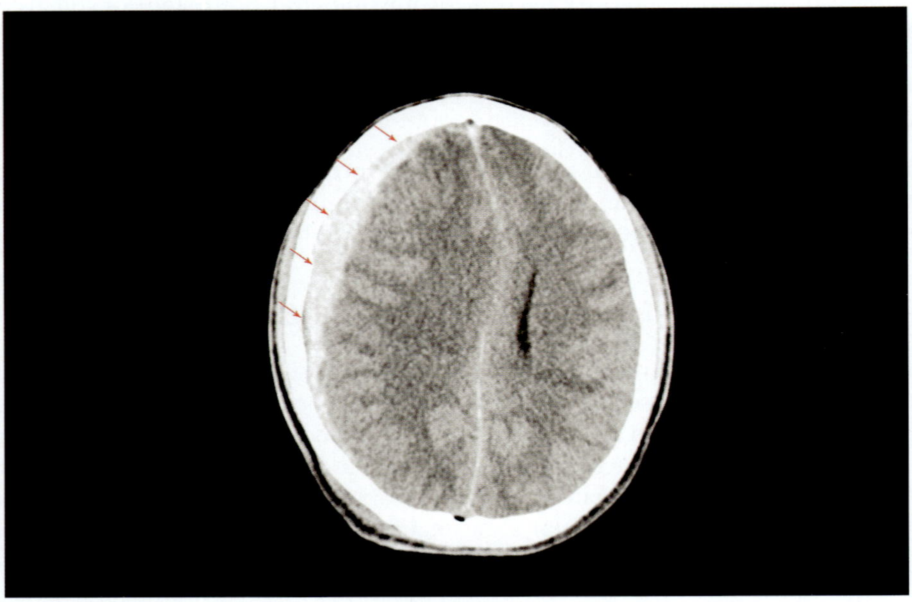

***Figure 13-2*** *CAT scan showing characteristic crescent shape (arrows) of a subdural hemorrhage. Note midline displacement. Subdural hemorrhage lies between the dura and arachnoid and is free to spread over the brain surface, unlike the epidural hemorrhage, which is constrained by the dura's attachment to bone.*

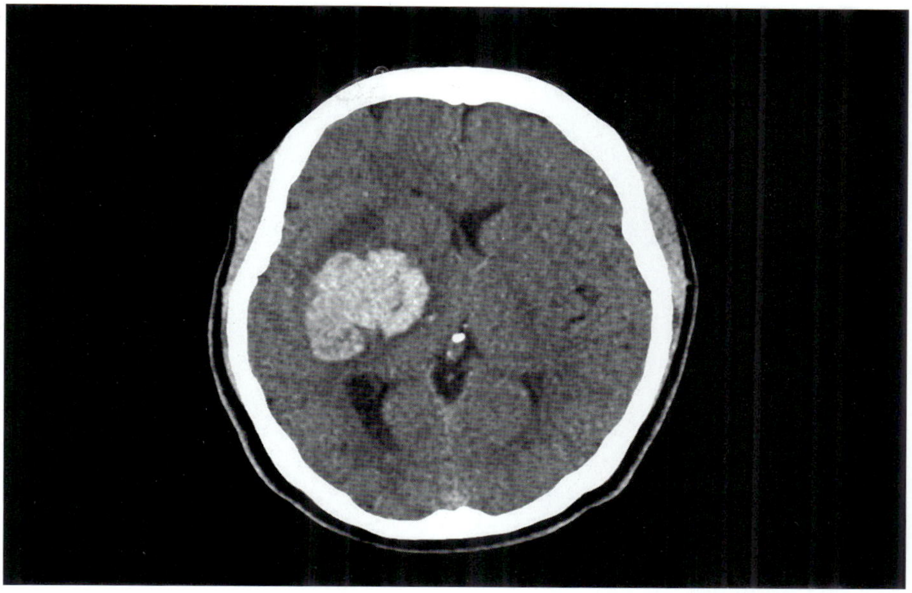

*Figure 13-3* *CAT scan showing intracerebral hemorrhage.*

## Magnetic Resonance Imaging (MRI)

Magnetic Resonance Imaging (MRI) examines the interior of the body without X-rays. It detects radiofrequency signals that are emitted by atomic nuclei after placing the patient in a strong magnetic field. This technique is a great advance over the CAT scan (which, like the MRI, shows the body as a series of sections) in that it allows much greater picture resolution as well as functional information about the tissue under examination. Since the MRI does not rely on radiation it can safely be repeated for serial follow-ups. It is better than the CAT scan for distinguishing gray from white matter in the brain and visualizing the posterior fossa and spinal cord. The MRI is used for diagnosing strokes, brain injuries, neurodegenerative diseases (e.g., Alzheimer's disease, Parkinson's disease, multiple sclerosis, amyotrophic lateral sclerosis), congenital brain defects, aneurysms, arteriovenous malformation, and brain and spinal cord tumors (**Fig. 13-4**). MRI is even more sensitive when enhanced with *gadolinium*. Gadolinium provides improved visualization of blood vessels, tumors, inflammation, demyelination (e.g., in multiple sclerosis), and infections. It helps differentiate between benign and malignant tumors based on their vascular supply and how they take up the contrast.

The downside of MRI is that it cannot be used on patients who have metallic objects in the body such as intracranial clips, certain pacemakers, cochlear implants, and intraocular metallic foreign bodies. It also may be difficult to perform in patients who are morbidly obese or very claustrophobic (the patient is placed within a narrowly closed area for the test) or cannot lie still due to a significant movement disorder.

The CAT scan can be done more quickly than an MRI and is generally less expensive and more readily available. The CAT scan is better than the MRI for detecting acute intracranial hemorrhage due to stroke or trauma in the first 36 hours, but beyond 2–3 days, MRI is

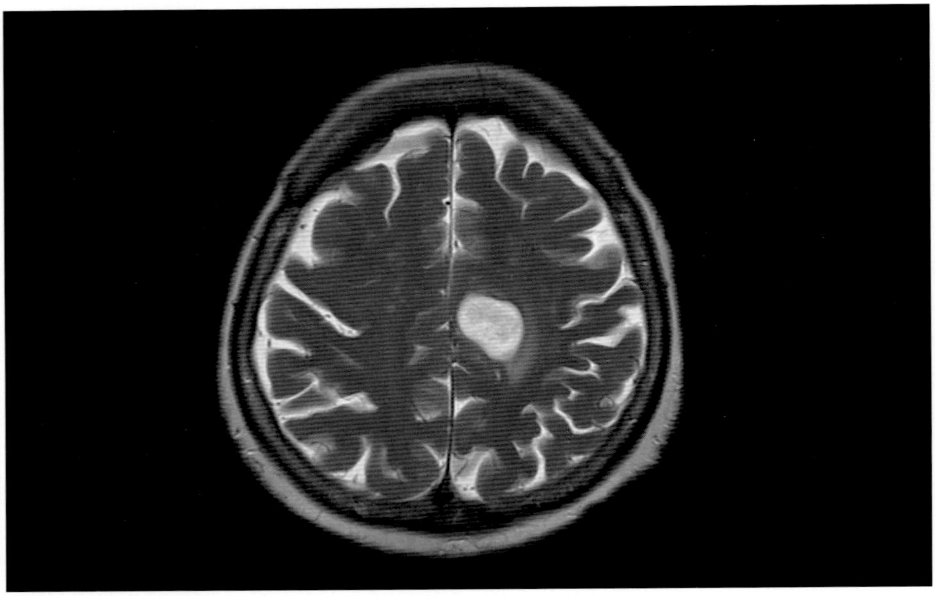

*Figure 13-4* *MRI showing brain tumor.*

better for detecting hematomas (local collections of blood that typically clot). The CAT scan may not show any abnormality within the first 12 hours, though, if the stroke is non-hemorrhagic. If the CAT scan is negative, an MRI, particularly with diffusion-weighted imaging, is more sensitive in detecting early stages of ischemic stroke. Both CAT scans and MRIs can tell if a lesion lies outside the brain, impinging on it, or lies within, infiltrating it.

**Diffusion-weighted MRI imaging (DWI)** measures the microscopic diffusion (Brownian movements) of tissue water molecules in the brain. It can detect acute ischemic stroke much earlier than the standard MRI, help diagnose tumors, and evaluate disease progression and response to treatment.

**Susceptibility-weighted MRI imaging (SWI)** is especially sensitive to molecules that distort the local magnetic field, making it useful to detect microhemorrhages or iron deposition.

**Diffusion Tensor MRI** applies the data from DWI to show the 3D shape of the diffusion. It shows white matter tracts and can be used preoperatively, for instance, to distinguish normal white matter paths from tumor. It also is used to assess the extent of brain matter pathology that affects white matter, such as multiple sclerosis, traumatic brain injury, stroke, and neurodegenerative diseases.

**T1-weighted MRI** makes water appear dark, and fat (like myelin) bright, useful for visualizing the normal brain anatomy, particularly differences between white and gray matter.

**T2-weighted MRI** (**Fig. 13-5**) makes water appear bright, and fat, which has low water content, darker, highlighting areas of edema, inflammation, or infection.

**FLAIR MRI** (**Fig. 13-6**) specifically suppresses the bright signal from cerebrospinal fluid (CSF), making it easier to detect abnormalities in the brain that are next to CSF, e.g., periventricular lesions in multiple sclerosis.

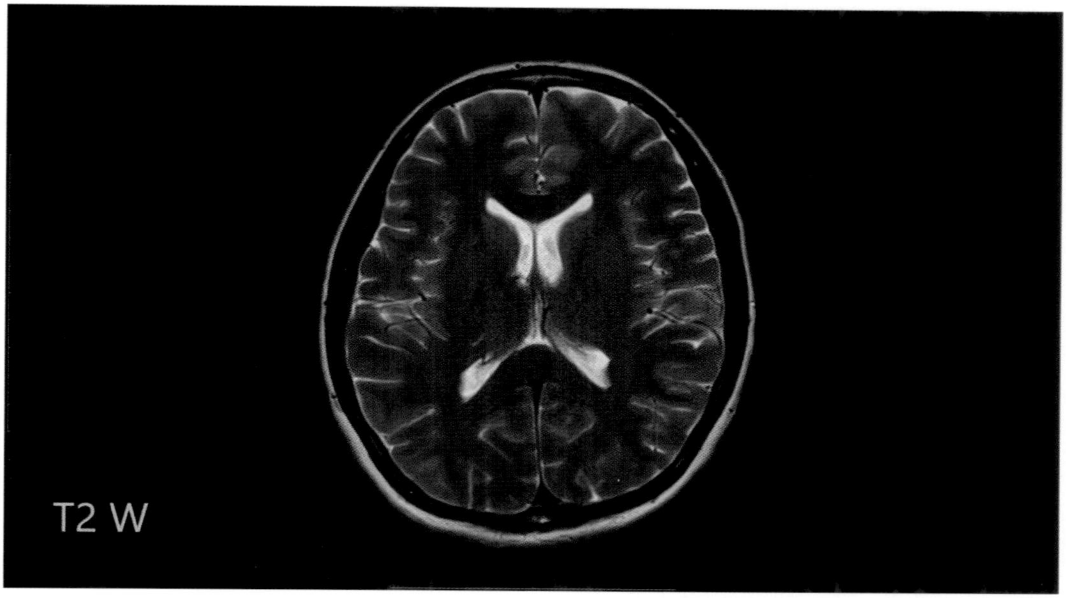


*Figure 13-5* *T2-weighted MRI. Note highlighted brightness of the ventricular cerebrospinal fluid.*

**Magnetic Resonance Angiography (MRA)** is a type of MRI that excels at examining arteries and veins, particularly following contrast injection into a vein. It can detect blood flow problems, blocked blood vessels, damage to vessel walls (e.g., dissection), aneurysms, and AV malformations, without the invasive use of catheters or radiation.

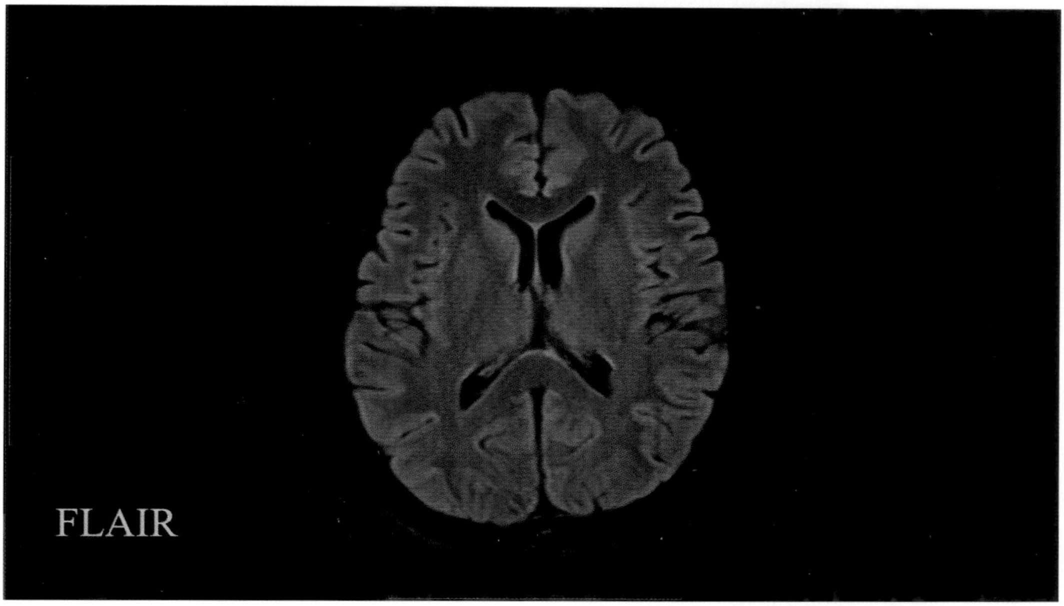


*Figure 13-6* *FLAIR MRI. Note suppressed brightness of the ventricular cerebrospinal fluid.*

**Functional MRI (fMRI)** uses the same scanner as a regular MRI, but it looks at brain function, not just structure. The patient is instructed to do certain exercises during the scan. The exercises increase the activity in specific areas of the brain, which then have increased blood flow and oxygenation, and which light up on the image, providing a measure of function. fMRI is used for brain mapping before surgery for epilepsy, tumors, or vascular malformations to avoid damaging essential brain areas during the operation. It is also used to study brain function in a variety of neurological disorders, both before and after treatment.

## Positron Emission Tomography (PET) And Single Photon Emission Computed Tomography (SPECT)

Positron Emission Tomography (PET) and Single Photon Emission Computed Tomography (SPECT) use radioactive tracers to examine cerebral metabolism and blood flow (**Fig. 13-7**). They are used to investigate dementias and certain cerebrovascular

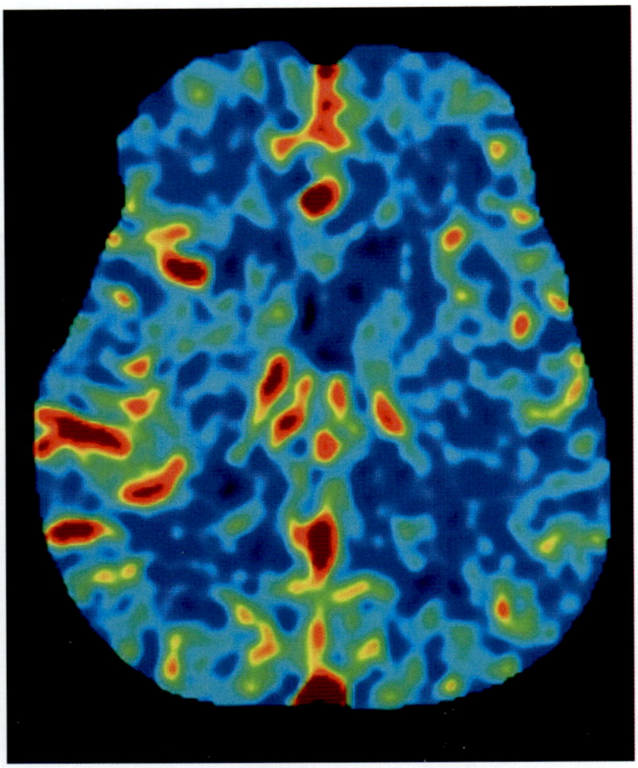

***Figure 13-7*** *PET scan of brain. Red indicates areas of high brain activity, particularly useful in comparing one side of the brain with the other (brain damage shows areas with reduced metabolic activity), monitoring disease progression, and evaluating treatment effectiveness.*

diseases and brain tumors, as well as to localize epileptic lesions. The PET scan can help distinguish the dementia of Alzheimer's disease from other dementias and help distinguish Parkinson's disease from progressive supranuclear palsy, a movement disorder that has certain similarities to Parkinson's disease. It can also help detect Huntington's disease in its early phases. The PET and SPECT scans differ in the radiotracers that they use. The PET scan detects positrons (from a labeled derivative of glucose [fluorodeoxyglucose]), while the SPECT scan detects gamma rays (e.g., from technetium-99m, iodine-123, or gallium-67). Unlike standard CT and MRI scans, PET and SPECT can also provide metabolic and functional information. In general, PET scans provide higher spatial resolution than SPECT scans, but tend to be more expensive and less widely available.

**Magnetoencephalography (MEG***)* detects magnetic fields produced by neural activity. It can be used to map brain function, e.g., in pre-surgical planning for epilepsy surgery.

## Imaging Techniques That Use Light

**Functional Near-Infrared Spectroscopy (fNIRS)** is a non-invasive method that uses light to measure brain activity. It can be used to measure surface blood flow and oxygenation in response to neural activity.

**Diffuse Optical Tomography (DOT)** is a non-invasive technique that analyzes the propagation of near-infrared light to examine blood flow in soft tissues, as inside the brain. It can construct 3D spatial maps of total hemoglobin concentration and blood oxygen saturation. It can also use fluorescent molecules that emit detectable photons. Although the spatial resolution is low, DOI can be used to provide information about brain function.

**Event-Related Optical Signaling (EROS)** uses infrared light to measure changes in the optical scattering properties of neurons in the cerebral cortex. Unlike DOT, which examines blood flow, EROS provides a direct measure of localized neuronal activity with a higher resolution than an EEG. The technique, though, is limited by reduced penetration into the head.

## Cranial Ultrasound

**Cranial Ultrasound** is done on infants to evaluate brain structure. It can only be done until the infant is about 14 months old, since ultrasound cannot scan through bone. It can detect abnormalities in brain development, brain injury, meningitis and encephalitis, hydrocephalus, bleeding in the brain or ventricles, and masses in the brain. It can also be used to guide the placement of needles. It is harmless, inexpensive, and can be done at bedside.

## Angiography

Angiography involves the injection into the arterial system of a contrast material that will outline the vascular system on X-ray (**Fig. 13-8**). This can reveal whether blood vessels

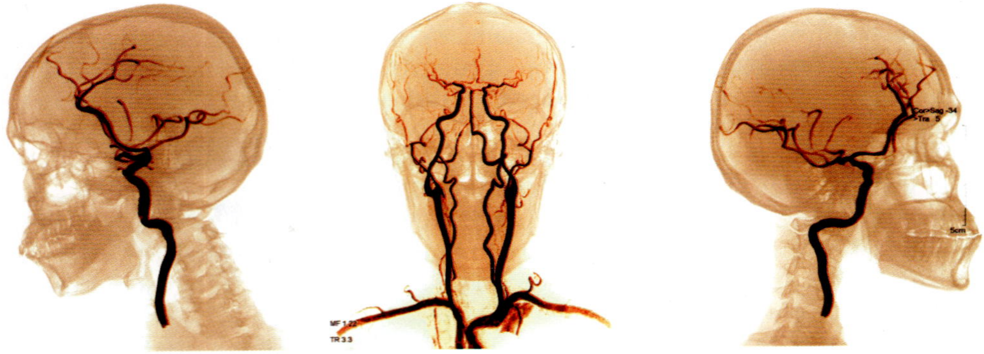

***Figure 13-8*** *Brain angiogram.*

are displaced (as may occur with tumors or hemorrhage), of abnormal pattern (as occurs in certain tumors, arteriovenous malformations, and aneurysms), occluded, or leaking. There is about 0.2% to 0.5% risk of developing a stroke from an angiogram, but the technique allows visualization of the continuity of cerebral vessels, which is difficult with the standard CAT or MRI scan alone. CT or MRI angiograms are options.

# 14

# Other Neurologic Tests

## Spinal Tap (Lumbar Puncture)

Spinal fluid is extracted from the lumbar cistern of the spinal canal and subjected to various analyses. Spinal fluid pressure is recorded at the time of extraction. Normal CSF opening pressure is 6-25 cm H2O in adults. The fluid itself is normally clear. It may contain excessive white cells and bacteria in infection; red cells (or **xanthochromia**, a yellowish color from breakdown of red blood cells) in subarachnoid hemorrhage; tumor cells; elevated proteins in tumors, hemorrhage, infections, and other conditions; and decreased sugar with bacterial infection. India ink applied to the fluid may outline cryptococcal organisms on microscopic exam. The fluid may also be cultured or submitted for more sophisticated analysis (e.g., **immunoelectrophoresis** – e.g., an elevated gamma globulin may be found in multiple sclerosis and in neurosyphilis).

A lumbar puncture (LP) is often ordered for:

- Suspected meningitis (fever + headache + neck stiffness)
- Suspected subarachnoid hemorrhage ("worst headache of my life")
- To rule out multiple sclerosis (young person with neurologic symptoms)

When NOT to do an LP:

Signs of increased intracranial pressure (papilledema, focal neurologic signs). Focal signs are a red flag for a possible mass lesion or unequal intracranial pressures. Doing an LP in that context can precipitate catastrophic brain herniation, so neuroimaging, e.g., a CAT scan, must rule out unsafe conditions first.

## Blood Tests

Blood tests that can be useful in neurologic diagnosis include:

**Complete Blood Count (CBC):** Can detect infections, inflammation, anemia, and other hematologic conditions responsible for fatigue, weakness, or cognitive disability

**Electrolytes and Kidney Function Tests:** Abnormal electrolytes can cause confusion, muscle weakness, seizures, and other neurologic deficits.

**Liver Function Tests:** Can detect hepatic encephalopathy

**Thyroid Function Tests:** Abnormal thyroid function may be responsible for myopathy, neuropathy, and cognitive problems.

**Glucose Levels:** Hypoglycemia or hyperglycemia may be responsible for alteration of consciousness or seizures.

**Vitamin B12 and Folate Levels:** Deficiency of B12 or folate can cause peripheral neuropathy and cognitive dysfunction.

**Inflammatory Markers (ESR, CRP):** Can suggest systemic infection or inflammation

**Autoimmune Antibodies:** May be present in a number of neurologic diseases (e.g., lupus, Sjögren's syndrome, autoimmune encephalitis)

**Infectious Disease Markers:** E.g., for HIV, syphilis, Lyme disease

**Toxicology Screen**: For therapeutic or non-therapeutic drugs

## Urine Tests

**Urinalysis:** E.g., for dehydration, proteinuria, hematuria, infections

**Urine Toxicology Screen:** For drugs and toxins

**Urine Metabolic Screen**: E.g., for porphyria, aminoacidurias, hyperammonemia

**24-Hour Urine Collection**: Can detect heavy metal poisoning (e.g., lead, mercury) that can cause neuropathy and other neurologic problems.

## Myelography

In this older technique, a liquid contrast material is injected directly into the lumbar subarachnoid space. This serves to outline on x-ray the spinal canal (and higher regions if the patient is tilted). Abnormalities of the spinal cord, intervertebral discs, or brain stem can be seen. This procedure has largely been replaced by CAT scans and MRI.

## Electroencephalography (EEG)

Although useful in localizing a lesion within the brain, the EEG has largely been supplanted in this regard by the CAT scan and MRI. The main use of the EEG is in the diagnosis of epilepsy (**Figs. 14-1** and **14-2**). **Magnetoencephalography (MEG)** senses the magnetic fields that neurons produce as opposed to the electrical signals that an EEG detects. It can better localize brain activity than the EEG.

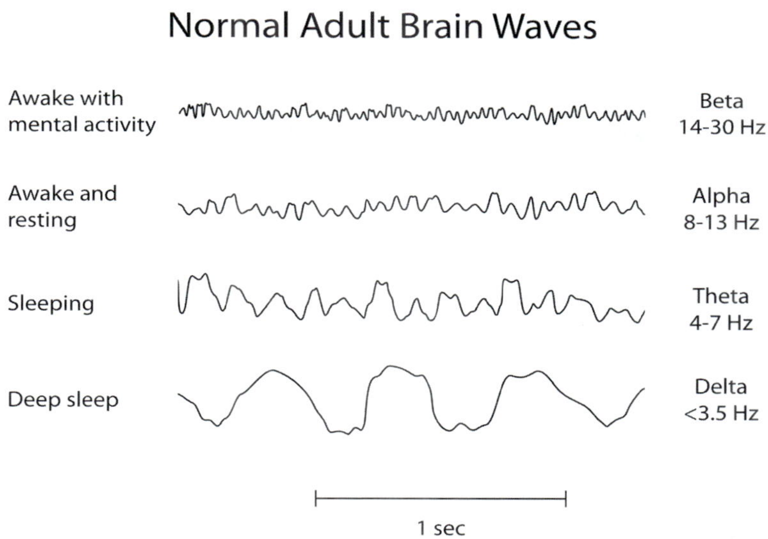


***Figure 14-1*** *Normal EEG patterns. Brain waves tend to be fastest when the subject is most alert.*

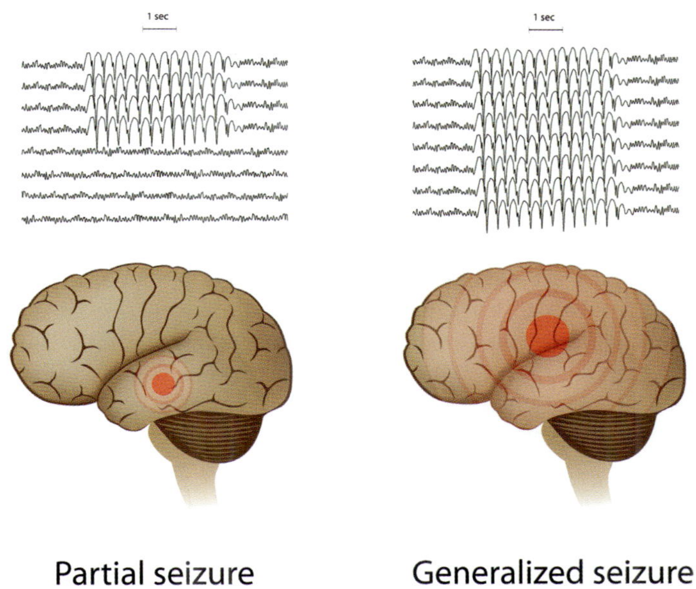


***Figure 14-2*** *EEG pattern in epilepsy.*

## Electromyography (EMG) And Nerve Conduction Studies (NCS)

EMG provides information about the electrical activity of muscles. Nerve conduction studies provide information about the speed and strength of nerve signals as they travel through nerves. EMG and NCS can help diagnose peripheral nerve disorders (e.g., peripheral neuropathy, carpal tunnel syndrome, Guillain-Barré syndrome, radiculopathy), muscle disorders (e.g., muscular dystrophy, myopathies, muscle atrophy), and neuromuscular junction disorders (e.g., myasthenia gravis, Lambert-Eaton Myasthenic Syndrome).

## Evoked Potentials

Evoked potentials (EPs) measure the electrical activity in the brain in response to a specific stimulus. **Visual evoked potentials** measure the response to specific visual stimuli and can help evaluate problems that affect the visual pathways, e.g., multiple sclerosis and optic neuritis. **Auditory evoked potentials** can help evaluate hearing loss. **Somatosensory evoke potentials** evaluate sensory pathways that convey touch sensation. Sometimes subtle changes of disease can be detected with EPs even before the symptoms are noticeable and can allow earlier treatment. EPs can also be used to monitor disease progression or improvement, as well as localize the part of the sensory pathway that is affected.

## Muscle And Nerve Biopsy

Muscle biopsy can sometimes help diagnose muscular dystrophies, inflammatory myopathies, metabolic muscle disease, and myasthenia gravis. Nerve biopsy can help diagnose peripheral neuropathies, vasculitic neuropathies, infectious conditions that affect the peripheral nerve, and amyloid neuropathy.

## Cognitive And Neuropsychological Tests

Tests of cognitive function, such as orientation, attention, calculation, recall, language, verbal fluency, visuospatial abilities, and executive function, can be administered by a neurologist, but are also administered by other professionals, including psychologists, neuropsychologists, psychiatrists, occupational therapists, speech-language pathologists, and trained co-workers. These tests focus on various aspects of cognition and can be used individually or as part of a battery of cognitive tests. They include:

- Mini-Mental State Examination (MMSE)
- Montreal Cognitive Assessment (MoCA)
- Trail Making Test (TMT)
- Wechsler Adult Intelligence Scale (WAIS)
- Wechsler Memory Scale (WMS)
- Boston Naming Test (BNT)
- Verbal Fluency Tests (VFTs)

- Clock Drawing Test (CDT)
- Rey-Osterrieth Complex Figure Test (ROCF)
- Wisconsin Card Sorting Test (WCST)

There are numerous kinds of tests in neurology. Rather than opting for a shotgun approach and ordering everything, the practitioner, with experience, should be able to select among the tests, prioritizing for testing those diagnoses that are more probable, more serious if missed, and more likely to lead to an effective remedy

# 15

# Neurologic Treatments

The neurologist accesses a variety of therapies, pharmacologic and otherwise, which are described in greater detail throughout the rest of the book. Although some procedures are performed by the neurologist, others are referred to the surgeon once the neurologist has made the diagnosis.

## Pharmacologic Treatments

- Antiepileptic drugs
- Analgesics and anti-inflammatory drugs for pain and inflammation
- Disease-modifying therapies for multiple sclerosis and other immune-mediated disorders
- Antiplatelet agents and anticoagulants for stroke prevention
- Anticholinergics and dopamine agonists for Parkinson's disease
- Cholinesterase inhibitors for Alzheimer's disease and other dementias
- Antidepressants, anxiolytics, and antipsychotics
- Other disease-specific agents

## Procedures

- Surgery for tumors, intracranial bleeds, hydrocephalus, epilepsy, herniated discs, spinal stenosis, and nerve compression
- Deep Brain Stimulation for Parkinson's disease, essential tremor, and dystonia

- Neurovascular surgery for stroke, aneurysms, and arteriovenous malformations
- Pain management: nerve blocks, epidural injections, medication pumps for chronic pain
- Intrathecal (within the CSF space surrounding the spinal cord) drug delivery for severe spasticity and pain
- Vagus nerve stimulation for epilepsy
- Neuromodulation techniques: Transcranial magnetic stimulation for depression and certain types of pain
- Gene therapy and stem cell therapy for certain genetic and degenerative disorders

## Rehabilitation

- Physical therapy
- Occupational therapy
- Speech and language therapy
- Lifestyle changes and supportive care: diet and exercise; cognitive-behavioral therapy and psychotherapy for mental health problems; support groups and counseling

The treatment should not be worse than the disease.

# Part III. Neurologic Presentations

There are hundreds of diseases in neurology. The chapter titles represent the way that the patient presents to the practitioner, with emphasis on the more common, treatable conditions.

# 16

# Headache

**Figure 16-1** lists the key causes of headache. Some are **primary** (e.g., migraines, tension headaches, cluster headaches, trigeminal neuralgia), since they are the main problem and not symptomatic of another condition. There are many headaches that are **secondary** to other medical conditions.

When to Worry:
EMERGENCY HEADACHES (Get help NOW):

- "Worst headache of my life": Subarachnoid hemorrhage (SAH) until proven otherwise
- Headache + fever + neck stiffness: Meningitis
- Sudden severe headache: Could be SAH, aneurysm
- Headache + confusion/weakness: Mass lesion, stroke

URGENT HEADACHES (Same day evaluation):

- New headache pattern in older patient: Rule out temporal arteritis
- Headache + visual changes: Rule out increased intracranial pressure
- Progressive headaches getting worse: Rule out mass lesion

NON-URGENT HEADACHES (Outpatient):

- Typical migraine pattern: Primary care or neurology
- Tension-type headaches: Supportive care
- Stable chronic headaches: Routine follow-up

*FIGURE 16-1. CAUSES OF HEADACHE*

**Primary Headache Disorders**
Tension Headaches
Migraine Headaches
Cluster Headaches
Trigeminal Neuralgia
Hemocrania Continua
Ice Pick Headache

**Secondary Headache Disorders**
Subarachnoid, Subdural, or Epidural Hemorrhage
Vascular Problems (Stroke, Transient Ischemic Attack, CNS vasculitis)
Infections (e.g., meningitis, encephalitis)
Dental or Jaw Problems
Sinusitis
Brain Tumor
Medication Overuse
Caffeine Withdrawal
Excess Alcohol Consumption (hangover)
Environment (weather, altitude, exposure to chemicals or pollutants)
Substance Use or Withdrawal
Angle Closure Glaucoma
Genetic Predisposition
Sleep Disorders
Allergic Rhinitis
Lupus
Rheumatoid Arthritis
Granulomatosis with Polyangiitis
Head Injury
Eye Strain
Physical Exertion
Hormonal Changes
Pseudotumor Cerebri
High Blood Pressure
Dehydration
Diet and Nutrition
Psychological Factors (stress; anxiety; personality traits)
Occipital Neuralgia
Nummular Headache
Orgasmic Headache
Primary Exercise Headache
Spontaneous Intracranial Hypotension Headache
Posterior Reversible Encephalopathy Syndrome (PRES)
Tolosa-Hunt Syndrome
Long COVID

Headache Red Flags:

- New or different
- Sudden / severe
- With fever
- With neurologic signs
- In patients > 50 years old

## Tension Headache

Tension headaches are the most common headache. They present as dull, non-pulsating pain that typically affects both sides of the head, often described as a tight band around the head or pressure on the forehead or temples.

### Diagnosis of Tension Headache

**Medical History**: Information should include a detailed medical history, including the frequency, duration, and characteristics of the headache, as well as anything that may trigger or worsen them (such as stress, poor posture, eyestrain, fatigue, overuse or withdrawal from caffeine or alcohol, teeth grinding, dehydration, certain foods, or skipped meals). Tension headaches can last for 30 minutes to a week and occur episodically. Generally, the pain is mild to moderate, rather than severe. Unlike migraines, tension headaches do not typically have associated symptoms like nausea, vomiting, or sensitivity to light and sound.

**Physical Examination**: Assess for signs of tension or muscle tenderness in the head, neck, and shoulders. Not everyone with muscle tension has tension headache, and not everyone with tension headache has muscle spasm. The reason for the condition may be more complex, involving alterations in brain chemistry. Confirm that the general neurological exam is normal.

**Imaging studies** (e.g., MRI or CT scan) are not usually necessary for diagnosing tension headaches unless there are concerning symptoms or signs of another underlying condition.

### Treatment of Tension Headache

**Over-the-Counter (OTC) Medications**: Mild tension headaches can often be managed with over-the-counter pain-relievers such as *acetaminophen (Tylenol), ibuprofen (Advil, Motrin)*, or *aspirin*. **Prescription Medications**: For more severe or frequent tension headaches, prescription medications may include muscle relaxants, tricyclic antidepressants (e.g., *amitriptyline*) or selective serotonin reuptake inhibitors (SSRIs), which may work by modulating the levels of neurotransmitters in the brain such as serotonin, norepinephrine, and dopamine, which play a role in regulating pain perception, mood, and stress response.

**Physical Therapy**: Massage, stretching exercises, and posture correction may help relieve muscle tension and reduce the frequency or severity of tension headaches.

**Stress Management Techniques**: Relaxation exercises, deep breathing, biofeedback, cognitive-behavioral therapy (CBT), and mindfulness-based stress reduction may help reduce tension.

**Lifestyle Modifications**: Improving sleep hygiene, staying hydrated, and avoiding triggers such as excessive caffeine or alcohol intake may help prevent tension headaches.

**Alternative Therapies**: Some individuals find relief from tension headaches with complementary and alternative therapies such as acupuncture, chiropractic manipulation, herbal supplements (e.g., *feverfew* or *butterbur*), aromatherapy, or dietary changes.

**Botox Injections**: *Onabotulinumtoxin A (Botox)* injections, approved for the preventive treatment of chronic migraine, may also be effective for some individuals with chronic tension headaches.

## Migraine Headache

Migraine headache is characterized by recurrent episodes of moderate to severe headache, often accompanied by other symptoms such as nausea, vomiting, and sensitivity to light and sound. It is usually unilateral and throbbing and can last several hours to several days. The frequency varies and the headaches may recur up to several times a month. Some people may experience an *aura* that precedes the headache. This can involve visual disturbances, sensory changes, or other neurological symptoms that typically develop over several minutes and may last up to an hour. Not everyone with migraine experiences an aura. Some people (the author is one of the lucky ones) may experience just the aura (e.g., scintillating scotoma moving laterally from the center of the visual field in each eye over about 20 minutes), without the headache. Migraine is believed to result from the dilation of blood vessels and activation of pain pathways.

### *Diagnosis of Migraine Headache*

There is no specific test for migraines. Migraine diagnosis mainly relies on the patient's history and ruling out other causes of headaches.

**Medical history** should include detailed documentation of the headache features, triggers, frequency, duration, and associated symptoms. Migraines commonly switch sides of the head in different attacks. Headaches that are always on the same side, particularly if they are worsening, should increase suspicion of a different cause.

**Neurological Examination**: To determine any coinciding neurological deficits

**Diagnostic Tests**: While not typically required for diagnosis, imaging (MRI or CT scan) and other tests may be conducted to rule out secondary causes of headache when other signs raise suspicion of another cause.

### *Treatment of Migraine Headache*

Treatment strategies for migraines include *abortive* treatment to relieve symptoms while having an attack and *preventive* treatment aimed at reducing the frequency and severity of attacks.

Abortive Treatment:

**NSAIDs**: *Ibuprofen*, *naproxen*, or *aspirin* often help for mild to moderate migraines.

**Triptans**: *Sumatriptan*, *rizatriptan*, and others are first-line treatments for moderate to severe migraines or when NSAIDs are ineffective. They stimulate serotonin receptors in the brain and are vasoconstrictors. By causing vasoconstriction, they help reduce the dilation of blood vessels that occurs during migraine. They also are anti-inflammatory and block brain pain pathways. Triptans are contraindicated in patients with cardiovascular disease due to the vasoconstriction, which may include blood vessels of the heart.

**Ergot Alkaloids**: Less commonly used today, vasoconstrictors like *ergotamine* (derived from the ergot fugus) are available for certain patients.

**Anti-Nausea Medication**: For those experiencing nausea or vomiting, medications like *metoclopramide* can help.

**CGRP (Calcitonin Gene-Related Peptide) Antagonists**: Newer classes of drugs such as *atogepant, ubrogepant* and *rimegepant* (CGRP receptor antagonists), given orally, or monoclonal antibodies against CGRP (*erenumab, fremanezumab, galcanezumab, eptinezumab*), given as monthly injections, have revolutionized headache medicine especially for frequent migraines. The newer CGRP antagonists (*ubrogepant, rimegepant*) provide alternatives for patients who can't use triptans due to cardiovascular disease. CGRP is a neuropeptide found in the nervous system and blood vessels. It is believed to be involved in the transmission of pain signals, release of inflammatory mediators, and promotion of vasodilation. Traditional options remain important: beta-blockers (propranolol), anticonvulsants (topiramate), and antidepressants (amitriptyline).

It is important to note that using acute migraine medications >10 days per month can cause rebound headaches that worsen the overall pattern.

Preventive Treatment:

**Beta-blockers** (e.g., *propranolol*) and calcium channel blockers (e.g., *verapamil*) to prevent excessive vasodilation, among other possible mechanisms

**Anticonvulsants** (e.g., *topiramate, valproate*) can help by stabilizing abnormal neuronal electrical activity and neurotransmitter balance that may be involved in migraines.

**Antidepressants** (e.g., *amitriptyline*) can help by modulating levels of serotonin and norepinephrine involved in pain processing.

**Botox Injections**: *Onabotulinumtoxin A* is approved for chronic migraines. Treatment involves multiple injections around the head and neck every 12 weeks. It is believed to help by relaxing muscles and modulating pain signaling.

**Lifestyle Modifications**: Adequate sleep schedule, hydration, regular meals, limited caffeine and alcohol intake, exercise, stress management, and avoidance of triggers play important roles in management. Although caffeine, through vasoconstriction, can help alleviate migraine pain in some patients, it may trigger migraines in others who are individually sensitive.

**Supplements**: Magnesium, riboflavin (vitamin B2), and coenzyme Q10 have been shown to reduce migraine frequency in some patients.

**Alternative therapies** include acupuncture, behavioral therapies (cognitive-behavioral therapy, biofeedback, relaxation techniques), herbal remedies (*feverfew, butterbur*), essential oils (*peppermint, lavender*), mindfulness and meditation, yoga, physical therapy, and chiropractic.

Migraine vs Tension Headache:

MIGRAINE:

- One-sided (but can be both)
- Throbbing / pulsating

- Nausea / vomiting
- Light / sound sensitivity
- Lasts 4-72 hours
- Family history often positive

TENSION:

- Both sides (band-like)
- Pressure / tightness (not throbbing)
- No nausea / vomiting
- No light / sound sensitivity
- Lasts 30 minutes to days
- Stress-related

Bottom line: If headache has nausea + light sensitivity = probably migraine

## Cluster Headache

Cluster headaches are a severe form of headache with recurrent episodes of intense dull pain on the same side of the head, usually around the eye or temple. These headaches occur in clusters or cycles, often lasting for weeks to months, followed by periods of remission. They usually last about 15 minutes to 3 hours but can occur up to 8 times a day during a cluster period. Tension headaches are often bilateral; migraines are more commonly unilateral and not always on the same side; cluster headaches more commonly recur on the same side. While stress is a common trigger for tension headaches, migraines and cluster headaches may be triggered by alcohol or certain foods.

### Diagnosis of Cluster Headache

**Medical History**: Ask about the frequency, duration, and characteristics of the headaches, as well as any associated symptoms such as tearing of the eyes, nasal congestion, or restlessness, which commonly occur in cluster headaches.

**Physical Examination**: May reveal pupil constriction, red, watering eye, eyelid drooping, runny nose or facial sweating on the affected side

**Imaging studies** (e.g., MRI or CT scan) are not usually necessary for diagnosing cluster headaches unless there are red flags of another underlying condition.

### Treatment of Cluster Headaches

**Acute Treatment**:

**Oxygen Therapy**: Inhalation of 100% oxygen through a mask can rapidly relieve acute cluster headache attacks, partly due to vasoconstriction.

**Triptans**: Subcutaneous *sumatriptan* or intranasal *zolmitriptan* (for rapid relief) is effective for aborting acute cluster headaches. These medications, which cause vasoconstriction and inhibit the release of neurotransmitters involved in pain signaling, may be used if oxygen therapy is not available or not effective.

**Intranasal Lidocaine**: May be used as an alternative to triptans for aborting acute cluster headache attacks, particularly in individuals who cannot tolerate triptans

**Preventive Treatment**:

***Verapamil***, a calcium channel blocker, is considered a first-line preventive treatment for cluster headaches. It is believed to modulate neural excitability and neurotransmitter release in the brain. It is typically started at a low dose and gradually titrated up to an effective dose to prevent cluster headache cycles.

**Corticosteroids**: Oral corticosteroids such as *prednisone* may be used as a bridge therapy during the initial phase of preventive treatment with verapamil or during acute cluster headache cycles to provide rapid relief. Corticosteroids have anti-inflammatory effects and cluster headaches may have an autoimmune component.

***Lithium***, which may modulate neurotransmitter systems involved in pain processing, can be used as an alternative or adjunctive preventive treatment for cluster headaches, particularly in individuals who do not respond to or cannot tolerate *verapamil*.

***Topiramate***, an anticonvulsant medication, may be considered as a second-line preventive treatment for cluster headaches in individuals who do not respond to or cannot tolerate *verapamil* or *lithium*.

**Other Treatments**:

**Nerve Blocks**: Occipital nerve blocks or sphenopalatine ganglion blocks may provide temporary relief for acute cluster headache attacks.

**Neuromodulation**: Occipital nerve stimulation or deep brain stimulation targeting the hypothalamus may be considered in individuals with refractory cluster headaches who do not respond to conventional treatments.

## Trigeminal Neuralgia

Trigeminal neuralgia is a chronic pain condition that affects the trigeminal nerve (CN5). The patient experiences sudden, severe electric shock pains that radiate along the trigeminal nerve distribution, typically on one side of the face. It may be caused by compression or irritation of the trigeminal nerve by a blood vessel, tumor, cyst, or arteriovenous malformation; trauma; demyelination from multiple sclerosis; or degenerative changes with aging. It may be idiopathic.

### *Diagnosis of Trigeminal Neuralgia*

**Physical Exam**: In some patients there may be sensory abnormalities such as numbness, tingling, or hypersensitivity in the affected facial area; decreased blink reflex (from interruption of the blink reflex arc that involves CN5 and CN7); twitching in the face; or trigger points that elicit pain. Otherwise, there are no specific diagnostic tests.

### *Treatment of Trigeminal Neuralgia*

**Medications:**

- **Anticonvulsants** such as *carbamazepine (Tegretol), oxcarbazepine, gabapentin,* or *pregabalin* are often first-line treatment. They stabilize cell membranes and decrease impulse transmission along the trigeminal nerve.

- **Muscle relaxants**, e.g., *baclofen*, may reduce muscle spasms, when used concurrently with anticonvulsants.
- **Tricyclic antidepressants**, e.g., *amitriptyline (Elavil)* may help relieve pain and facilitate sleep.

**Surgical Procedures:**

- **Microvascular Decompression:** A surgical procedure behind the ear inserts a small pad to relieve pressure from an offending blood vessel pressing on the trigeminal nerve.
- **Percutaneous Procedure:** Percutaneous balloon compression, glycerol rhizotomy (nerve root severing), radiofrequency rhizotomy, and stereotactic (gamma knife) radiosurgery are procedures used to damage the trigeminal nerve and block pain signals.
- **Neurectomy:** A portion of the trigeminal nerve may be removed in refractory cases but carries the risk of permanent facial numbness along the nerve distribution.

**Botulinum (Botox) injections** in areas of the face that experience pain may be used to block the release of neurotransmitters involved in pain transmission.

**Alternative Therapies:** Some patients report relief from alternative therapies, such as acupuncture, chiropractic care, or biofeedback.

## Hemicrania Continua

Hemicrania continua is a rare primary headache disorder characterized by continuous head pain, always on the same side of the head, which may involve the frontal, temporal, or occipital regions. It fluctuates in intensity and is associated with autonomic symptoms on the side of the headache. It may have to do with a neurochemical imbalance in pain processing or blood flow regulation in the brain, with a possible genetic predisposition. Environmental factors such as stress, sleep disturbances, hormonal fluctuation, and dietary factors may trigger an attack. Hemicrania continua differs from cluster headache in being continuous rather than presenting in episodic clusters. Autonomic symptoms are usually less pronounced than in cluster headaches. Also, hemicrania continua responds well to *indomethacin*, while cluster headache doesn't.

### *Diagnosis of Hemicrania Continua*

**History**: Note the frequency, duration, and characteristics of the headaches, as well as any associated symptoms such as autonomic features (e.g., tearing of the eye, nasal congestion, or eyelid drooping, and facial flushing or sweating, all on the side of the headache) and response to medications.

**Physical Exam**: Test for tenderness to touch on one side of the head (typically not a significant symptom), as well as any associated autonomic symptoms (ptosis, red eye, lacrimation, nasal congestion, facial sweating, miosis, or eyelid swelling) on the affected side.

**Diagnostic Tests**: There are no specific diagnostic tests for hemicrania continua. Diagnosis is mainly based on clinical criteria, unilateral head pain of moderate intensity or greater, with exacerbations of severe pain and at least one autonomic symptom, in addition to a successful response to *indomethacin*.

## *Treatment of Hemicrania Continua*

**Indomethacin**: *Indomethacin*, a nonsteroidal anti-inflammatory drug (NSAID), is the first-line treatment for hemicrania continua. Most individuals with hemicrania continua experience complete resolution of headache symptoms within hours to days of starting *indomethacin* therapy. A positive response to *indomethacin* is considered diagnostic for hemicrania continua. *Indomethacin,* apart from its anti-inflammatory effects, can inhibit vasodilation and may modulate the release of neurotransmitters involved in pain. It also penetrates the blood-brain barrier well.

**Other Medications**: In individuals who do not respond to or cannot tolerate *indomethacin*, treatment may include other NSAIDs, corticosteroids, or medications commonly used for other types of primary headaches, such as triptans.

**Long-Term Management**: Once hemicrania continua is confirmed, long-term treatment with *indomethacin* is usually necessary to maintain symptom control.

**Lifestyle Modifications**: Lifestyle modifications such as maintaining regular sleep patterns, managing stress, staying hydrated, and avoiding triggers may help reduce the frequency and severity of hemicrania continua attacks.

**Supportive Therapies**: Some individuals with hemicrania continua may benefit from physical therapy, relaxation techniques, or biofeedback to help manage pain and improve overall quality of life.

# Ice Pick Headache

Ice pick headaches (primary stabbing headaches) are characterized by recurring episodes of brief stabbing or jolting electric shock-like pains that occur spontaneously and typically last for a few seconds to a minute. The pain may be unilateral or bilateral. The condition may relate to dysfunction of the trigeminal nerve or the pain processing areas with the brain. It differs from trigeminal neuralgia in that the pain is broader in distribution than in trigeminal neuralgia. Also, there is no particular trigger such as a light touch to the face, as in trigeminal neuralgia. Ice pick headaches tend to occur more frequently than episodes of trigeminal neuralgia, sometime several times in the day, and as shorter episodes.

## *Diagnosis of Ice Pick (Primary Stabbing) Headaches*

**Medical History**: Ask about the frequency, duration, and characteristics of the headache. Ice pick headaches have a sudden onset, short duration, and a stabbing or jolting quality. It typically does not respond to the same medication as trigeminal neuralgia.

**Physical Examination**: A physical examination is performed to assess for signs of other neurological conditions that may cause headaches. Ice pick headaches are typically not associated with other neurological abnormalities.

**Diagnostic Tests**: There are no specific diagnostic tests for ice pick headaches. Diagnosis is primarily based on the clinical history of brief, stabbing or jolting pains occurring spontaneously in the absence of any other underlying neurological condition.

## *Treatment of Ice Pick Headaches*

**Acute Treatment**: Ice pick headaches are generally self-limited and do not usually require specific treatment. However, if the pain is severe or bothersome, over-the-counter pain relievers such as nonsteroidal anti-inflammatory drugs (NSAIDs) or *acetaminophen* may be used to alleviate symptoms. This differs from the treatment of trigeminal neuralgia, which often responds to anticonvulsants, such as *carbamazepine (Tegretol), oxcarbazepine,* and *gabapentin.*

**Preventive Treatment**: In some cases, if ice pick headaches are frequent or disruptive, preventive treatments may be considered such as anticonvulsants (e.g., *gabapentin, topiramate*), tricyclic antidepressants (e.g., *amitriptyline, nortriptyline*), beta blockers (e.g., *propranolol, nadolol*), or calcium channel blockers (e.g., *verapamil*).

**Lifestyle modifications** include relaxation exercises, meditation, or yoga to manage stress; maintaining regular sleep patterns and adequate hydration; avoiding potential triggers, such as foods to which the individual may be sensitive; environmental factors; or activities that may precipitate the headaches.

# Temporal Arteritis

Temporal arteritis (*giant cell arteritis; GCA*), is a type of vasculitis that mainly affects the arteries in the head, particularly the temporal arteries, which can lead to severe complications, such as vision loss if not promptly treated.

## *Diagnosis of Temporal Arteritis*

**History**: Symptoms can include new-onset headache, often localized to the temporal regions; scalp tenderness; jaw claudication (pain in the jaw when chewing); visual disturbances (such as temporary or permanent vision loss or double vision); fatigue; weight loss; and fever.

**Physical Exam**: Palpation of the temporal arteries is painful and may reveal thickening, nodularity, or a decreased pulse.

**Lab Tests**:

- **Erythrocyte Sedimentation Rate (ESR)** and **C-Reactive Protein (CRP)**, when elevated, suggest inflammation but are not specific to temporal arteritis.
- **CBC** may show normochromic, normocytic anemia (anemia of inflammation).

**Temporal Artery Biopsy** is considered the gold standard for diagnosis, where a small segment of the temporal artery is surgically removed and examined for inflammation and giant cells. However, a negative biopsy does not rule out GCA due to the patchy nature of the disease.

**Imaging**:

- **Ultrasound**: Can show a halo sign around the temporal artery, indicating inflammation
- **MRI** or **CT Angiography**: For assessing the involvement of larger vessels
- **PET Scan**: May be used to detect inflammation in larger vessels not accessible by ultrasound

## *Treatment of Temporal Arteritis*

Treatment focuses on quickly reducing inflammation to prevent complications, especially vision loss. Immediate treatment with high-dose **corticosteroids**, such as *prednisone*, is standard to rapidly decrease inflammation. The dose is gradually reduced based on symptoms and inflammation markers (ESR and CRP levels). Long-term treatment may be necessary, often lasting 1-2 years or longer. Patients on long-term corticosteroids are monitored for side effects, such as osteoporosis, diabetes, hypertension, and increased risk of infections. Calcium and vitamin D supplements, along with bisphosphonates, may be recommended to prevent bone loss.

**Adjunctive Therapy**: For patients who cannot tolerate corticosteroids or, as a steroid-sparing strategy, other immunosuppressive drugs like *methotrexate* or *tocilizumab* (an IL-6 receptor antagonist) may be used.

Visual symptoms require urgent evaluation by an ophthalmologist.

## Subarachnoid Hemorrhage

Subarachnoid hemorrhage commonly presents as a sudden, severe headache (*thunderclap headache*), often described as "the worst headache in my life." It usually results from rupture of an **aneurysm** in the region of the Circle of Willis. This **arterial bleeding** enters the subarachnoid space, which extends around the brain stem and spinal cord down into the neck and back. The headache is often characterized as severe pain in the back of the head, neck, and back.

### Diagnosis of Subarachnoid Hemorrhage

**Imaging**: The situation is an emergency. Non-contrast head **CT scan** is the first-line imaging modality because of its rapidity and sensitivity in showing acute hemorrhage within the first 24 hours.

**Lumbar Puncture**: If the CT scan is inconclusive, lumbar puncture can reveal red blood cells or *xanthochromia*, a yellowish discoloration of the CSF arising from breakdown of hemoglobin within the first few hours of the bleed.

**CT angiography** can detect the presence of the aneurysm and its precise location, information needed for surgical intervention.

### Treatment of Subarachnoid Hemorrhage

**Coil embolization** is minimally invasive, often preferred to **surgical clipping** of the aneurysm, since it does not require opening the skull. Soft platinum coils are positioned in the aneurysm sac; the coils induce clotting inside the aneurysm, decreasing the chance of aneurysm bleeding and rupturing. However, the feasibility of doing coil embolization depends on the size, shape, and location of the aneurysm, as well as the patient's clinical status. In the case of **intracerebral hemorrhage**, treatment of a large hemorrhage may require hematoma evacuation via craniotomy.

## Subdural Hemorrhage

Subdural hemorrhage is a **venous hemorrhage**. It results from the tearing of bridging veins between the brain and dural sinuses, generally resulting from head trauma, sometimes even minor head trauma in the elderly. Apart from headache, the patient may experience other neurologic symptoms, sometimes acutely over hours, depending on the size and location of the hemorrhage. These may include confusion, memory loss, weakness or sensory loss on one side of the body, speech difficulty, visual problems, seizures, and gait problems. While symptoms may occur acutely, they may develop slowly with chronic enlargement of the hematoma over weeks to months.

### Diagnosis of Subdural Hemorrhage

The neurologic exam provides some index of the extent of brain injury. CAT scan of the head is the standard initially because of its ability to visualize bleeding. Subdural hemorrhage commonly appears crescent-shaped on CAT scan (**Fig. 13-2**). MRI may be used for further evaluation, particularly with chronic subdurals.

### Treatment of Subdural Hemorrhage

Small subdurals without significant symptoms may only need close observation with repeat imaging. Antiepileptic drugs may be prescribed for seizure prevention. For larger subdurals, surgery may be recommended, either by burr hole trephination, craniotomy to remove the hematoma, or placement of a subdural drain to remove fluid over time.

## Epidural Hemorrhage

Epidural hemorrhage is an **arterial** hemorrhage, resulting most commonly from a skull fracture, particularly involving the middle meningeal artery, which runs in the skull bone. Fracture commonly occurs at the **pterion**, the lateral H-shaped landmark indicating the junctions of frontal, sphenoid, parietal, and temporal bones. Commonly, the patient loses consciousness briefly but may do so again several hours after awakening as the bleeding continues. While X-ray can reveal the fracture, CAT scan is better, since it can confirm not only the fracture but the hemorrhage and its dimensions. Epidural hemorrhage commonly appears biconvex (lens-shaped) on CAT scan (**Fig.13-1**). MRI can be useful when the diagnosis is not clear.

It is important to keep the patient under close observation, which may be all that is necessary along with repeat imaging if the hematoma is small. Larger hematomas may require burr holes to reach and drain the hematoma, or a craniotomy, in which part of the skull bone is separated to remove the hematoma. The patient may receive anticonvulsants to guard against seizures, as well as analgesics.

## Meningitis And Encephalitis

**Meningitis** is an inflammation of the meninges, the membranes around the brain. It can be caused by viral, bacterial, fungal, and parasitic infections, reaction to certain medications (e.g., NSAIDs, trimethoprim-sulfamethoxazole, certain immunosuppressants), metastatic disease, or, occasionally, an autoimmune condition. Symptoms in viral meningitis may be milder than those of bacterial meningitis. **Encephalitis** is an inflammation of the brain. It is often caused by viral infections but can also result from bacterial infections or as an autoimmune disease.

Patients with meningitis or encephalitis often have overlapping symptoms due to the close anatomical and functional relationships of the brain and the meninges. Both meningitis and encephalitis can present with:

**Headache**: Often severe

**Fever**

**Nausea and Vomiting**

**Stiff Neck**: A classic sign, making it difficult to bend the neck forward, more common in meningitis, as the meninges cover the brain and spinal cord

**Photophobia:** More common in meningitis, due to inflammation of the meninges around the optic nerve

**Weakness or Loss of Motor Skills**: More prominent in encephalitis due to involvement of the brain.

**Problems with Speech or Hearing**: Difficulty understanding or producing speech, or hearing loss, more common in encephalitis due to brain involvement that may extend to the auditory nerve or inner ear

**Confusion or Altered Mental Status**: More common in encephalitis due to brain involvement

**Seizures**: More common in encephalitis due to brain involvement

**Drowsiness or Coma**: More common in encephalitis due to brain involvement

## *Diagnosis of Meningitis and Encephalitis*

**Clinical Examination:** Initial assessment of symptoms such as fever, neck stiffness, *Kernig's sign*, *Brudzinski's sign*, headache, altered mental status, and seizures

**Lumbar Puncture:** Can detect inflammation, pathogens, autoimmune antibodies, and other abnormalities. **Figure 16-2** shows cerebrospinal (CSF) differences between bacterial, viral, fungal, and parasitic infections. Other tests, e.g., Gram stain, India ink preparations

**FIGURE 16-2. CSF FINDINGS IN INFECTIONS**

| Organism | CSF Appearance | WBC Count | Protein | Glucose | Culture | Examples |
|---|---|---|---|---|---|---|
| **Bacterial** | Cloudy if high WBC count | High (often >1000 cells/$\mu$L); mainly neutrophils | Very elevated | Decreased (bacteria eat glucose) | Pos. for bacteria | Pneumococcus, Meningococcus |
| **Viral** | Usually clear | Moderately elevated (10-500 cells/$\mu$L); mainly lymphocytes | Slightly elevated or normal | Normal or slightly decreased | Neg. for bacteria | Enteroviruses, Herpes simplex virus |
| **Fungal** | Clear or slightly cloudy | Elevated, but usually less than bacterial; mainly lymphocytes | Elevated | Decreased | Fungal cultures may be pos. | Cryptococcal meningitis, Coccidioidomycoses |
| **Parasitic** | Clear or cloudy | Variable, may show eosinophilia | May be elevated | Usually normal | Neg. for bacteria | Toxoplasmosis, Neurocysticercosis (pork tapeworm) |

(for fungal infections like Cryptococcus) and antigen/antibody or PCR tests can further narrow down the cause of infection.

**Blood tests** can identify the presence of bacteria or viruses (e.g., PCR for bacterial or viral DNA; latex agglutination test for certain bacteria) that might have caused the infection; specific tests for antibodies associated with autoimmune encephalitis.

**Imaging**: CT or MRI is done before lumbar puncture (LP) if increased intracranial pressure or brain abscess is suspected, due to the risk of brain herniation with LP.

### Treatment of Meningitis and Encephalitis

Treatment depends on the cause:

**Bacterial Meningitis:** Needs urgent antibiotic therapy, often started empirically before causative bacteria are identified.

**Viral Meningitis:** Generally milder than bacterial meningitis and often treated with supportive care, such as hydration and pain management. Specific antiviral medications may be used for certain viruses like herpes simplex virus.

**Fungal and Parasitic Meningitis:** Treated with specific antifungal or antiparasitic medications.

Corticosteroids may be given in certain cases of bacterial meningitis to reduce inflammation and prevent complications.

**Viral Encephalitis:** Antiviral therapy may be given for encephalitis caused by viruses like herpes simplex (e.g., *acyclovir*). Unfortunately, rabies encephalitis (from rabies virus transmitted by the saliva of infected animals) is almost always fatal once symptoms appear. Pre-exposure prophylaxis with rabies vaccine, and post-exposure prophylaxis with wound cleaning, rabies immunoglobulin and rabies vaccine are highly successful if administered soon after exposure.

**Immunotherapy:** For autoimmune encephalitis, treatments may include steroids, intravenous immunoglobulins (IVIG), or plasmapheresis (removes autoantibodies) to modulate the immune response.

**Supportive Care:** Manage fever, ensure proper hydration, and treat seizures or other complications. Both encephalitis and meningitis may require intensive care support, especially in severe cases or when there are complications such as seizures, severe swelling, or breathing difficulties. The long-term management might include rehabilitation services, such as physical therapy, occupational therapy, or speech therapy, depending on the residual effects of the illness.

## Angle Closure Glaucoma

In angle closure glaucoma, which is typically unilateral, there is a sudden blockage of aqueous humor exit from the eye, due to the collapse of the angle between the iris and trabecular meshwork of the eye (**Fig. 16-3**). The angle appears shallow on examination. Apart from acute, severe pain, the vision in the eye may be blurred due to clouding of the cornea. The eye, as palpated through the upper eyelid, feels rock hard in comparison with the normal eye because of increased ocular pressure. The pupil is mid-dilated and non-reactive to light, and the conjunctiva may be red.

(**Ultrasound biomicroscopy** or anterior segment **optical coherence tomography** can provide detailed images of the anterior segment and help confirm the diagnosis.)

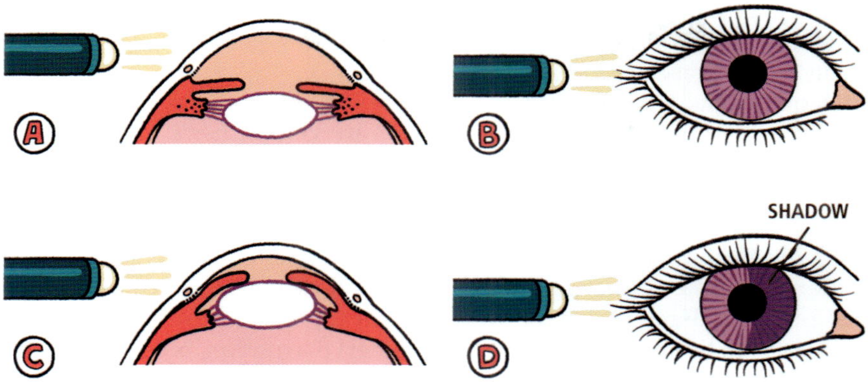


*Figure 16-3* *Assessing the depth of the anterior chamber in angle closure glaucoma. A and B, normal angle. C and D. Shallow chamber with narrow angle. A shadow forms because of the curved positioning of the iris. (From Goldberg, S. and Trattler, W.* Ophthalmology Made Ridiculously Simple, *Medmaster)*

### Treatment of Angle Closure Glaucoma

In order to prevent optic nerve damage, the patient should be immediately referred to the ophthalmologist for more definitive treatment, as the condition is highly curable. In the meantime, intraocular pressure can be reduced quickly with an oral or IV **carbonic anhydrase inhibitor** (e.g., *acetazolamide*) or a **hyperosmotic agent** (e.g., *oral glycerin* or IV *mannitol*).

**Laser peripheral iridotomy** is the definitive treatment of angle closure glaucoma, since making a small hole in the iris allows aqueous humor to flow normally.

## Pseudotumor Cerebri

Pseudotumor cerebri is a condition with increased intracranial pressure of unknown cause, commonly seen in overweight women of childbearing age. The patient may present with headache, visual disturbances, and tinnitus. Retinal exam shows papilledema. Lumbar puncture reveals elevated CSF pressure with normal CSF composition. MRI or CT scans do not reveal any mass lesion or hydrocephalus. The treatment includes:

**Diuretics** (e.g., *acetazolamide, topiramate*) to reduce CSF production

**Migraine treatment** for headache

**Cerebrospinal fluid shunting** or **serial lumbar punctures** when medication does not sufficiently control symptoms.

## Other Types of Headache

**Sinusitis**, an inflammation of the tissue lining the maxillary, frontal, ethmoid, or sphenoid sinuses of the facial bones, can be caused by infections, allergies, air pollution, or structural problems. There may be nasal congestion and increased pain on pressing on the affected sinus. A CAT scan (better than an MRI for viewing bone) can provide detailed images of the sinuses. Nasal or sinus cultures can identify an infection, and allergy tests can determine if allergies are implicated. Treatment includes adequate hydration, decongestants, analgesics, antihistamines, nasal corticosteroids, saline nasal irrigation, and antibiotics where indicated. Allergy shots or endoscopic surgery to remove blockages may be advised in chronic cases.

**Occipital neuralgia**, like trigeminal neuralgia, involves sharp, stabbing, or electric shock-like pains that may have triggers, in this case certain head movements, whether turning or bending the neck. The condition may be caused by muscle tension, nerve entrapment, cervical spine disorders or head or neck trauma. The pain radiates from the base of the skull up the back of the head. Treatment may include analgesics, rest, heat or cold therapy, physical therapy, posture correction, and stress management.

**Nummular headache** is characterized by a round or elliptical "coin-shaped" area of pain, about 2-6 cm in diameter, on the back, side, or top of the head, on one or both sides. The cause is unclear, but may involve peripheral nerve irritation, muscle tension, changes in the central nervous system, or psychological or genetic predisposition. It can be treated with over-the-counter pain medication, tricyclic antidepressants, anticonvulsants, muscle relaxants, topical lidocaine or, sometimes, nerve blocks or botulinum toxin injections. Massage or stretching exercises or the scalp, neck and shoulders, cognitive-behavioral therapy, and stress management have helped some. Evidence is limited for acupuncture or nutritional supplements, such as magnesium, vitamin B2 (riboflavin), or coenzyme Q10.

**Orgasmic headache** ("sex headache") is a rare type of headache that occurs during sexual activity, typically at orgasm. It may last minutes to several hours. It is treated with over-the-counter pain medications, migraine medications, *indomethacin* taken before sexual activity, beta-blockers to reduce blood pressure, relaxation techniques, and gradual, relaxed sexual activity or altering of sexual positions that may trigger the headache.

**Primary exercise headache** occurs during or after physical exertion such as running or weightlifting. It is treated by adequate hydration, gradual warming up before exercise, gradual cooling down afterwards, and over-the-counter pain medications. *Indomethacin* may be effective when taken before physical activity but can be accompanied by gastrointestinal irritation with long-term use. Beta-blockers (e.g., *propranolol*) may be considered for their effect in reducing blood pressure and heart rate. Consider whether there may be certain triggers to the headache (e.g., heat, humidity, certain foods).

**Spontaneous intracranial hypotension headache** is mainly caused by leakage of cerebrospinal fluid. The headache worsens with upright posture and improves on lying down. There may also be neck stiffness, nausea, vomiting, or visual disturbances. CSF pressure is low ($<60$ mm $H_2O$). MRI can show thickening and enhancement of the dura mater (which may be from dilatation of dural blood vessels, as well as downward displacement of the cerebellar tonsils through the foramen magnum. Exam may show papilledema. MRI of the spine may show epidural fluid collections. Treatment can be conservative (bed rest, hydration, caffeine to reduce vasodilation, and analgesics. Corticosteroids (e.g., *prednisone*) can help reduce any inflammation around the leak; *acetazolamide* may be prescribed to reduce CSF volume and restore normal pressure gradients. An epidural blood patch, epidural fibrin glue injections, or direct surgical repair may be used to seal the leak.

**Posterior reversible encephalopathy syndrome (PRES)** is classically characterized by a combination of headache, altered mental status, seizures, visual disturbances, and MRI findings of edema mainly confined to the posterior regions of the brain (but can affect other brain regions). It is reversible with prompt diagnosis and treatment of its underlying cause, which may include entities as diverse as severe hypertension, immunosuppressive or chemotherapeutic medications, autoimmune diseases, electrolyte disturbances, infection, or toxins. It can be treated symptomatically with analgesics but mainly by addressing its underlying cause.

**Tolosa-Hunt syndrome** is a rare, typically recurrent disorder characterized by severe, unilateral periorbital headaches, often accompanied by weakness or paralysis of the eye muscles. It results from inflammatory granulomatous lesions of the cavernous sinus or posterior eye socket. It is proposed that the condition may be an autoimmune reaction to structures within the cavernous sinus. This leads to inflammatory granulomatous lesions that compress structures within the sinus, including the trigeminal nerve and nerves to the ocular muscles. Treatment typically involves corticosteroids or other immunosuppressive medications to reduce inflammation and diminish symptoms.

**Long COVID** is persistent symptoms following a COVID-19 infection, lasting more than 4-12 weeks after the acute illness. It may be experienced by as many as 10-30% of the general population. Common symptoms include headache, dizziness, fatigue ("brain fog") shortness of breath, chest pain or palpitations, sleep disturbances, anxiety, depression, loss of smell or taste, GI symptoms, and muscle and joint pain. The treatment is supportive; the headache is treated with standard migraine or tension-type headache medication.

Other secondary causes of headache, as listed in **Figure 16-1**, can largely be suspected and ruled out based on the patient's routine history, physical exam, and lab tests.

# 17

# Back Pain and Sciatica

Back pain has many causes, which can be classified in several ways:

**Musculoskeletal Causes of Back Pain**

- **Muscle or Ligament Strain**: Heavy lifting, sudden movement, or chronic overuse can strain back muscles and spinal ligaments.
- **Bulging or Ruptured Discs** can press on a nerve.
- **Arthritis**: Osteoarthritis, rheumatoid arthritis, ankylosing spondylitis, psoriatic arthritis, enteropathic arthritis, and gout can affect the lower back.
- **Spondylolisthesis**: A condition in which one vertebra slips forward over another one
- **Compression Fractures**: Typically related to osteoporosis, these can cause severe back pain.
- **Scoliosis**

**Neurological Causes of Back Pain**

- **Sciatica**: Sharp, shooting pain that radiates from the buttock down the back of one leg, caused by an impingement on the sciatic nerve by a herniated disc, spondylolisthesis (slipped vertebra), spinal stenosis, or muscle spasms in the buttocks.
- **Spinal Stenosis**: Narrowing of the spinal column that puts pressure on the spinal cord and nerves (**Fig. 17-2**).
- **Radiculopathy**: Compression, irritation, or injury to a spinal nerve root, causing pain, numbness, or weakness. This should be distinguished from a **peripheral neuropathy**, where there is something intrinsically wrong with the peripheral nerve, aside from compression, e.g., diabetes, infections, toxic exposures, inherited disorders.

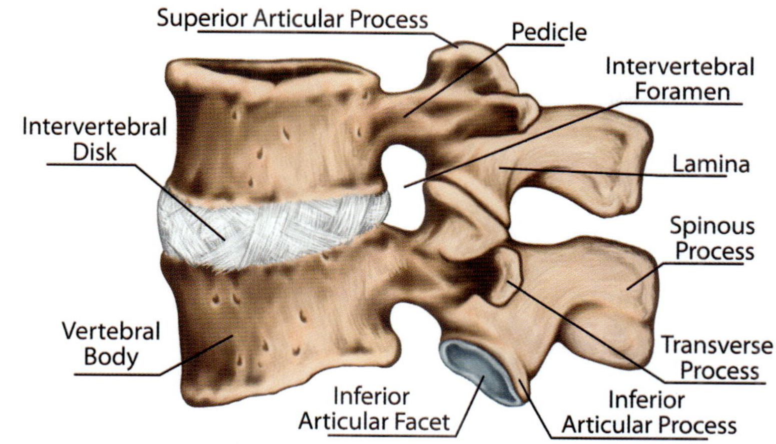


***Figure17-1*** *Vertebrae.*

- **Cauda Equina Syndrome**: Acute loss of function of the lower nerve roots of the spinal canal, leading to severe pain, bladder and / or bowel dysfunction, sexual dysfunction, potential motor weakness or lower motor neuron paralysis of one or both legs, and loss of sensation in the saddle area. **Conus medullaris syndrome**, which affects the lower end of the spinal cord (L1-L2 vertebra level), can present similarly, but with a mixture of upper and lower motor neuron signs since it involves the spinal cord as well as the nerve roots. Treatment may include surgical decompression (e.g., laminectomy or discectomy) or tumor removal if that is the cause.

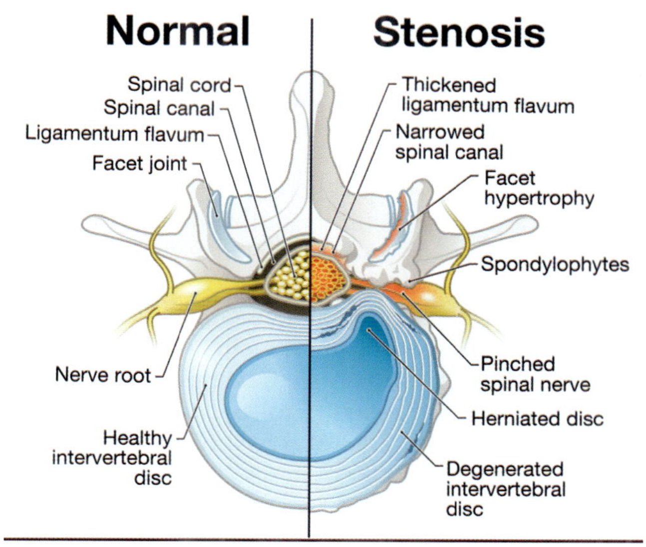


***Figure 17-2*** *Spinal stenosis. Narrowing of the spinal canal can occur through herniated discs, degenerative changes in the spine, thickened ligaments within the spine, trauma, bone spurs (spondylophytes) or congenital factors.*

### Infectious and Inflammatory Causes of Back Pain

- **Osteomyelitis**: Infection of the vertebrae
- **Discitis**: Infection in the discs between vertebrae
- **Pott's Disease**: An inflammatory disease of the spine caused by tuberculosis.

### Traumatic Causes of Back Pain

- **Injuries**: From falls, accidents, sports, resulting in fractures, sprains (ligament injury), and strains (muscle or tendon injury)

### Degenerative Conditions Causing Back Pain

- **Degenerative Disc Disease**: Wear and tear on the discs, causing pain
- **Facet Joint Dysfunction**: Wear and tear or arthritis affecting the vertebral facet joints, causing pain and stiffness

### Other Causes of Back Pain

- **Kidney Stones or Kidney Infection**: Can cause severe pain that is felt in the back, often very painful on tapping the painful area
- **Endometriosis**: Uterine lining tissue outside the uterus can cause pain that radiates to the back.
- **Fibromyalgia**: A condition that causes widespread musculoskeletal pain, including back pain
- **Tumors** on the spine or nearby structures can cause back pain.
- **Constipation**

### Psychological Factors

- **Stress** can cause or exacerbate back pain due to muscle tension.

*Diagnosis of Back Pain*

**History**: How long has the patient had the pain? What are the characteristics of the pain, along with any associated symptoms, such as radiculopathy, weakness, or sensory changes? What worsens or improves the pain? Is there a history of injury? What is the patient's occupation? How physically active is the patient? Moving around or sitting all day on the sciatic nerve at a desk, with poor posture or adequate chair support? Inquire about previous treatments and their result. Inquire about symptoms that may indicate systemic causes of back pain, such as fever (infection), weight loss (cancer, infection), or urinary problems (kidney stones, bladder infection).

**Physical Exam**: Note the posture, spinal alignment, and any obvious signs of injury. Check for tenderness, swelling, or other abnormalities, as well as range of motion to assess the spine's flexibility. Pain on straight leg raising 30-70 degrees suggests irritation or compression of the lumbar nerve roots (L5 or S1), as with a lumbar disc herniation and radiculopathy. Saddle anesthesia (loss of sensation in the areas that would touch a saddle on riding a horse) suggests a cauda equina or conus medullaris lesion, as would the report of urinary or fecal incontinence and decreased anal sphincter tone. Other neurologic defects might raise concern about spinal cord compression.

**Imaging**: If the pain is severe, persistent, or there are other concerning symptoms, imaging tests (X-ray, MRI, or CT scan) may be diagnostic. X-rays can reveal bone abnormalities, such as fractures, arthritis, or spinal alignment issues. MRI can evaluate soft tissues, including discs, ligaments, nerve root compression, spinal stenosis, spondylolisthesis, or tumors. CT is useful when MRI is contraindicated or not available and is particularly good in evaluating bony structures.

**Blood Tests**: Can detect markers of inflammation or infection that might suggest specific causes like ankylosing spondylitis or spinal infection

**Urine Tests:** If kidney stones or kidney infection is a consideration

**Neurological Tests**: Electromyography (EMG) and Nerve Conduction Studies (NCS) can help detect nerve damage and confirm the level of nerve involvement.

**Bone scan** is occasionally used to detect bone tumors or compression fractures from osteoporosis.

**Discography** involves injection of a contrast dye into a spinal disc to evaluate disc health.

Back Pain Red Flags:

EMERGENCY (Immediate surgery consult):

- Cauda equina syndrome: Back pain + loss of bowel/bladder control
- Progressive leg weakness + back pain
- Saddle anesthesia (numb buttocks/groin)

URGENT (Same day evaluation):

- New weakness in legs
- Severe pain not responding to usual measures
- Fever + back pain (possible infection)

ROUTINE (Outpatient management):

- Mechanical back pain without red flags
- Chronic back pain with stable symptoms
- Muscle strain type pain

Pearls:

1. Straight leg raise (pain shooting down leg = nerve irritation)
2. Reflexes (absent = nerve problem)
3. Strength testing (weakness = nerve compression)
4. Sensation (numbness in specific pattern = nerve root)

Most back pain is mechanical - focus on finding red flags.

### *Treatment of Back Pain*

The treatment of back pain varies based on the underlying cause and the intensity of the pain. Treatment options include:

**Conservative Management**: Initial treatment often includes rest, applying heat or ice, and over-the-counter pain relievers. Patients are also advised to stay active, avoiding activities that worsen the pain, practice good posture, and lose weight if it is excessive. Physical therapy can strengthen the muscles in the back and abdomen, improve flexibility, and increase spinal stability, which can help alleviate pain.

**Medications**:

- **Pain Relievers**: Over-the-counter pain relievers (NSAIDs or acetaminophen) are often recommended. In more severe cases, stronger prescription medications may be needed.
- **Muscle Relaxants**: If muscle spasms are a part of the pain syndrome
- **Nerve Pain Medications**: Medications like *gabapentin* or *pregabalin* may be prescribed for sciatic pain. These act by binding to specific sites on nerve cells to reduce the release of neurotransmitters involved in pain transmission.
- **Epidural Steroid Injections**: Corticosteroid injections into the epidural space can help reduce inflammation around the irritated nerve and temporarily relieve pain.
- **Antibiotics for Infection**: E.g., for osteomyelitis, discitis, or Pott's disease (spinal tuberculosis)
- **Assistive devices** include walking aids (canes or walkers) to provide support; supportive footwear; lumbar support cushions; standing desks; heating pads and ice packs; and back braces for short-term use. A **TENS** (Transcutaneous Electrical Nerve Stimulation) unit delivers low-voltage electrical currents to decrease pain by stimulating nerves through electrode pads placed on the skin.

**Surgery**: Surgery may be considered if conservative treatments fail and the pain is severe, or if there are significant neurological deficits like muscle weakness or loss of bowel or bladder control. Common surgical procedures include **discectomy** (removal of the herniated portion of a disc) and **laminectomy** (removal of part of the back of the vertebral bone that's pressing on the affected nerve) (**Fig. 17-1**). A **foraminotomy** may be done to enlarge the foramen where the nerve root exits (e.g., to remove *spondylophytes* [bone spurs]) (**Fig. 17-2**), to relieve pressure on the nerve. A **spinal fusion** joins two or more vertebrae together to stabilize the spine, sometimes with screws and rods. **Minimally invasive lumbar decompression** focuses on removing excess ligamentous tissue, to increase the space in the spinal canal in spinal stenosis. **Interspinous spacers** can be implanted between the vertebral spines to increase the space for the nerves, without removing vertebral bone or tissue.

**Alternative Therapies**: Some people find relief through acupuncture, chiropractic manipulations, or massage therapy, although the effectiveness of these treatments can vary.

# 18

# Weakness

Weakness can arise from problems in the central or peripheral nervous system, neuromuscular junction, muscle, or from systemic conditions (**Fig. 18-1**). After establishing *where* the problem lies through the history, physical exam, and tests, further testing can identify the specific cause and recommended treatment.

### *Diagnosis of Weakness*

Weakness can primarily originate within the central nervous system, peripheral nerves, neuromuscular junction, or muscle. It can also be a manifestation of systemic abnormality (e.g., electrolyte or endocrine disorders, infections, cardiac disease, alcoholism).

**History:** Distinguish whether the patient is describing true weakness or simply fatigue or sensory loss.

**Onset and Progression**: Ask about the onset (acute vs. gradual) and progression of the weakness. Certain neurological causes of weakness arise quickly, e.g., stroke, Guillain-Barré Syndrome, myasthenia gravis exacerbation, acute spinal cord injury. Others arise more gradually, e.g., amyotrophic lateral sclerosis (ALS), chronic inflammatory demyelinating polyneuropathy, muscular dystrophies, spinal muscular atrophy, and peripheral neuropathies. Some conditions (e.g., myasthenia gravis; multiple sclerosis) can have acute exacerbations as well as a more gradual course of progressive weakness.

Are there any associated symptoms such as muscle wasting or sensory changes?

**Distribution**: Is the weakness generalized or localized?

*Generalized weakness* occurs in:

- Guillain-Barré syndrome in later stages
- Myasthenia gravis and ALS in later stages

## FIGURE 18-1. CAUSES OF WEAKNESS

***Central Nervous System Causes of Weakness***

**Ischemic Stroke**

- Thrombosis (e.g., from hypercoagulable states, trauma, inflammation, dehydration, pregnancy, oral contraceptives, intravenous drug use, genetic factors)
- Embolic Stroke (e.g., blood clot release from atrial fibrillation, heart valve or other cardiac abnormalities, atherosclerosis, patent foramen ovale; fat, air bubble, or tumor fragment emboli)
- Systemic Hypoperfusion
- Atherosclerosis
- Small Vessel Disease
- Transient Ischemic Attack
- Carotid or Vertebral Artery Dissection

**Hemorrhagic Stroke**

- Aneurysm
- Arteriovenous Malformation
- Hypertension
- Carotid or Vertebral Artery Dissection
- Cerebral Amyloid Angiopathy (amyloid deposits can weaken blood vessel walls)

**Other Central Nervous System Causes of Weakness**

- Multiple Sclerosis
- Brain and Spinal Cord Tumors
- Traumatic Brain Injury
- Spinal Cord Injury
- Cerebral Palsy
- Amyotrophic Lateral Sclerosis
- Polio
- Leukodystrophies (degenerative diseases caused by genetic mutations that affect the myelin sheath in the brain and spinal cord)

***Peripheral Nervous System Causes of Weakness***

- Peripheral Neuropathy
- Guillain-Barré Syndrome
- Charcot-Marie-Tooth disease (a hereditary motor and sensory neuropathy that predominantly affects peripheral nerves)

***Neuromuscular Junction Causes of Weakness***

- Myasthenia Gravis
- Botulism
- Lambert-Eaton Myasthenic Syndrome (a rare autoimmune disorder with muscle weakness, often associated with small cell lung cancer)

***Muscle Causes of Weakness***

- Muscular Dystrophies
- Polymyositis (an autoimmune inflammatory disease affecting mainly proximal muscles)
- Dermatomyositis (similar muscle involvement as polymyositis, but with skin rash, different antibodies, and a higher risk of malignancies)
- Metabolic Myopathies (inability of muscles to adequately metabolize energy)
- Glycogen Storage Diseases
- Fatty Acid Oxidation Disorders
- Mitochondrial Myopathies
- Periodic Paralysis (a group of genetic disorders that cause muscle weakness at irregular intervals)
- Spinal Muscular Atrophy (a genetic disorder with progressive muscle weakness and atrophy)
- Statin Myopathy
- Malignant Hyperthermia (An inherited mutation that disrupts calcium regulation in skeletal muscle cells leads to an uncontrolled hypermetabolic response when exposed to triggering anesthetic agents.)

***Other Causes of Weakness***

- Infections
- Electrolyte Imbalances (e.g., hypokalemia, hyperkalemia, hypophosphatemia)
- Toxins (e.g., heavy metal poisoning, organophosphate poisoning from pesticides)
- Endocrine Disorders
- Heart Disease
- Diabetes
- Smoking
- Obesity
- High Cholesterol
- Excessive Alcohol Use
- Physical Inactivity

- Muscular dystrophies
- Polymyositis and dermatomyositis
- Chronic inflammatory demyelinating polyneuropathy (CIDP)
- Metabolic myopathies
- Spinal muscular atrophy
- Periodic paralysis
- Botulism
- Rhabdomyolysis

*Localized weakness* is more likely to occur with:

- Stroke or brain tumors
- Mononeuropathies (e.g., carpal tunnel syndrome; ulnar, radial, and peroneal nerve neuropathies)
- Spinal cord lesions (e.g., herniated disc, myelopathy)
- Motor neuron disease (e.g., early-stage ALS)
- Focal myositis
- Nerve root disorders (cervical or lumbar radiculopathy)
- Infections (e.g., polio)

Does it affect proximal, distal, or specific muscle groups?

*Proximal muscle weakness* is caused by:

- Certain muscular dystrophies (e.g., Duchenne Muscular Dystrophy, Becker Muscular Dystrophy)
- Metabolic myopathies (glycogen storage diseases, mitochondrial myopathies)
- Endocrine disorders (thyrotoxic myopathy, hypothyroid myopathy, Cushing Syndrome [cortisol effect], and steroid-Induced myopathy)
- Myasthenia gravis (ocular and proximal limb muscles)

*Distal muscle weakness* occurs with:

- Peripheral neuropathies (e.g., diabetic neuropathy, Charcot-Marie-Tooth Disease [progressive muscle weakness and atrophy in the distal limbs, foot deformities, such as high arches and hammer toes, and reduced sensation due to demyelination or axonal damage of peripheral nerves])
- Some forms of ALS may present initially with distal muscle weakness and later cause proximal weakness.
- Distal myopathies
- Some neuromuscular junction disorders (Lambert-Eaton Myasthenic Syndrome may initially present distally)
- Some neurologic diseases can affect both proximal and distal muscles, depending on the stage of the disease. Understanding where the weakness lies helps guide diagnostic tests, if needed, such as EMG, nerve conduction studies, muscle biopsy, and genetic testing.

**Exacerbating or Relieving Factors**: Information on what worsens or improves the weakness can provide clues to its etiology. For instance:

- The weakness in *myasthenia gravis* typically worsens with sustained use, improves with rest, and is better in the morning.

- Weakness improves with repeated use in *Lambert-Eaton Myasthenic Syndrome*.
- Changes in potassium intake (too much or too little) can exacerbate weakness in *periodic paralysis*.
- In *metabolic myopathies* (e.g., glycogen storage disease or mitochondrial myopathies), weakness may be exacerbated by exercise, fasting, illness, or certain dietary changes. Exercise testing can help confirm this.

**Medical History**: Past medical history, including any chronic illnesses, previous similar episodes, family history of neurological diseases, and medication use

**Physical Exam:**

- **Motor Exam**: Assessment of muscle strength and tone, including *rigidity* (resistance to passive movement of a limb at any speed) or *spasticity* (resistance to passive movement at higher speeds of movement), significant atrophy (more so than simple disuse), or the presence of muscle fasciculations. (Fasciculations by definition are visible twitching; fibrillations are not visible but are detectable with EMG.)
- **Sensory Exam**: Evaluation of tactile, pain, temperature, vibration, and proprioceptive sensation helps determine if there is a sensory component, which is more suggestive of a neuropathy rather than a myopathy.
- **Reflex Assessment**: Is there hyperreflexia (an upper motor neuron sign), hyporeflexia or areflexia (lower motor neuron signs)?
- **Coordination and Gait Tests**: Helps identify cerebellar involvement
- **Cranial Nerve Exam**: Although the focus is on weakness, one or more cranial nerve deficits places the lesion above the foramen magnum.

**Blood tests** can look for metabolic, inflammatory, or infectious causes. These include complete blood count, electrolytes, renal and liver function tests (impaired renal / liver function may lead to accumulation of toxic substances), thyroid function tests (hypothyroidism can be associated with myopathy; hyperthyroidism with tremors and muscle weakness), and specific markers, e.g., creatine kinase (elevations suggests muscle damage).

**Autoimmune panels** such as antibodies associated with multiple sclerosis, neuromyelitis optica (*Devic's disease*: inflammation and demyelination of the optic nerves and spinal cord, with vision loss and spinal dysfunction), myasthenia gravis, autoimmune encephalitis, or paraneoplastic neurological syndromes, can help confirm an autoimmune disease. Paraneoplastic syndromes are a group of rare disorders that are triggered by an abnormal immune system response to a cancerous tumor. Such syndromes can affect the nervous system, endocrine glands, skin, blood, and other organs.

PCR testing, antibody serology, or isolation of the virus from stool, throat, or CSF can confirm **polio**.

**Electrophysiological Studies**: Electromyography (EMG) and nerve conduction studies (NCS) can differentiate between nerve and muscle disorders.

**Imaging**: MRI of the brain or spinal cord can identify central lesions. MRI can also detect inflammation in muscles. Muscle and nerve ultrasound may be diagnostically useful by identifying structural changes or lesions in muscle or nerve.

**Specific Tests**: Depending on the suspected diagnosis, more targeted tests like genetic testing, muscle or nerve biopsy, or lumbar puncture might be necessary.

Weakness Patterns - Quick Assessment:

PATTERN 1: One Side of Body Weak

- Location: Brain (stroke, tumor)
- Clues: Face + arm + leg on same side
- Action: STROKE ALERT if sudden, urgent imaging if gradual

PATTERN 2: Both Legs Weak, Arms OK

- Location: Spinal cord
- Clues: "Level" where sensation changes, bowel/bladder problems
- Action: URGENT - spinal cord compression

PATTERN 3: Arms and Legs, Hands/Feet First

- Location: Peripheral nerves
- Clues: Glove/stocking pattern, diabetes history
- Action: Check blood sugar, B12, thyroid

PATTERN 4: Just Muscles Weak, No Numbness

- Location: Muscle or neuromuscular junction
- Clues: Gets worse with use (myasthenia), muscle pain
- Action: Neurology referral, check creatine kinase (CK)

Even Quicker Assessment:

- One side = Brain
- Both legs = Spinal cord
- Glove/stocking = Nerves
- Just weakness = Muscle

*Treatment of Muscle Weakness*

Treatment depends on the underlying diagnosis:

**Acute Management**: For some conditions, like Guillain-Barré syndrome or myasthenic crisis, immediate intervention in a hospital setting may be necessary.

**Chronic Management**: For chronic conditions, such as muscular dystrophies or neuropathies, treatment may involve physical therapy, occupational therapy, and medications to manage symptoms.

**Medications**: These may include immunosuppressants for autoimmune neuropathies, enzyme replacement for certain metabolic myopathies (e.g., glycogen storage disease type II), acetylcholinesterase inhibitors for myasthenia gravis.

Supportive treatments include those for pain, spasticity (e.g., oral *baclofen*, *tizanidine*, *diazepam* or *dantrolene* for muscle spasticity; *intrathecal baclofen* for severe spasticity; *botulinum toxin* injections into spastic muscles), and support for autonomic dysfunctions like orthostatic hypotension, gastroparesis, urinary retention, constipation, anhidrosis or hyperhidrosis, sexual dysfunction, or cardiac arrhythmias.

# Central Nervous System Causes of Weakness

## Stroke

A stroke (cerebrovascular accident; CVA) is a sudden interruption of blood supply to part of the brain, resulting in a neurological deficit, the nature of which depends on the affected area of the brain.

There are two main kinds of stroke:

- An **ischemic stroke**, where a thrombus or an embolus cuts off the blood supply. About 85% of strokes are ischemic.
- A **hemorrhagic stroke** (about 15% of strokes), where a blood vessel in the brain bursts, leading either to bleeding inside the brain (**intracerebral hemorrhage**) or bleeding between the brain and its surrounding membranes (**subarachnoid hemorrhage**).
- Stroke-like symptoms may also occur from pressure on the brain from a bleed under the dura (**subdural hemorrhage**) or between the dura and its surrounding bone (**epidural hemorrhage**), both commonly arising from head trauma. Subdural hemorrhage is a venous hemorrhage that arises from the tearing of veins that bridge the brain's surface and the dural sinuses. Epidural hemorrhage is an arterial hemorrhage, commonly resulting from a skull fracture that involves tearing of the middle meningeal artery, which runs within the skull bone.

Arterial dissection (e.g., vertebral or carotid artery) can lead to an ischemic or hemorrhagic stroke. Rarely, chiropractic manipulation of the neck can result in a vertebral artery dissection.

It is critical to determine whether a stroke is ischemic or hemorrhagic since this significantly affects treatment. Anticoagulants may be used in an ischemic stroke but are contraindicated if there has been an arterial bleed.

Venous hemorrhage is not necessarily a contraindication to anticoagulation when it is due to cerebral venous thrombosis. Then, anticoagulation may be considered depending on the size and cause of the bleed, to prevent further thrombus formation and help resolve the clot.

*Diagnosis of Stroke*

**History** should include:

- **Time of Onset.** The exact timing is important since the administration of thrombolytic agents has only a narrow time window (typically within 4.5 hours).
- **Symptom Progression.** Did the symptoms arise suddenly, progressively worsen, or fluctuate? Ischemic strokes commonly have a sudden onset, while hemorrhagic stroke symptoms might progress more slowly as the bleeding continues. If the symptoms improved, the condition might be a stroke mimic, such as a seizure, migraine, transient ischemic attack, or metabolic problem, e.g., hypoglycemia.
- **The current symptoms**, whether localized weakness, sensory loss, difficult speaking, coordination, or visual problems helps localize the lesion.
- **Past history** should be obtained of any strokes or transient ischemic attacks (TIAs). A history of TIAs raises the risk of stroke, as does a history of diabetes, cardiovascular disease, dyslipidemia, sickle cell, coagulopathies, or vasculitis.
- Note any medications the patient is taking, such as anticoagulants or antiplatelet drugs (e.g., aspirin).

- Is there a family history of stroke or cardiovascular disease?
- A history of smoking, alcohol excess, recreational drugs, or unhealthy diet may raise the risk of stroke.
- Potential stroke mimics include hypoglycemia (check the glucose immediately); seizure with postictal paralysis (Todd's paralysis); migraine with aura; Bell's palsy; and functional neurologic disorders. These require different treatments.

**Physical Exam:** The neurologic exam can help localize the stroke. If there are accompanying sensory symptoms such as sensory or visual loss, this not only indicates that the weakness is not of muscular origin, but also helps pinpoint where in the nervous system the lesion may lie, such as the cerebrum, brain stem, or spinal cord.

### Imaging:

- **Non-contrast CT scan of the head** can differentiate between ischemic and hemorrhagic stroke. It is essential for ruling out hemorrhage before thrombolytic therapy. CT is more sensitive than an MRI in detecting acute hemorrhage within the first 24-48 hours. It is often the first test done and is quicker and often more available than an MRI. Non-contrast CT rules out hemorrhage but may be normal in early ischemic stroke. CT angiography identifies large vessel occlusions requiring thrombectomy. Advanced imaging techniques such as CT perfusion or MRI enable personalized stroke treatment by identifying areas of the brain that are at risk but still salvageable. Treatment can be offered to those with favorable imaging, even outside traditional time limits - safely and with potential for meaningful recovery. And one can avoid treatment in patients with large infarcts and little salvageable tissue (due to high risk of hemorrhage or futility).

- **MRI of the brain with diffusion weighted imaging (DWI)** is more sensitive than conventional MRI in detecting early ischemic changes, often with minutes to a few hours after symptom onset. It can also help determine the age of a stroke, since DWI lesions evolve over time.

- **CT angiography** and **MR angiography** are used for assessing the cerebral vasculature, identifying occlusions and aneurysms, and planning potential endovascular interventions.

- **Vascular Evaluation** with **Carotid Doppler Ultrasound** can evaluate for significant stenosis or occlusion in the carotid arteries. **Transcranial Doppler** can assess intracranial arterial patency. **Echocardiography** can identify cardiac sources of emboli, such as atrial fibrillation.

Non-contrast CT scan is also excellent for diagnosing subdural or epidural hemorrhage in the acute stage. MRI is often preferred later, since its resolution is better than a CT scan and can provide information about the age of the hemorrhage and any underlying brain injury. Sometimes, MRI can detect a small amount of blood that might be missed by CT.

**Cerebral venous thrombosis (CVT)** can present with symptoms resembling those of arterial stroke. It is diagnosed with MRI venography or CT venography. Blood tests for risks of deep vein thrombosis (DVT) can look for clotting disorders, autoimmune diseases, and infections.

Quick stroke assessment:

- **FAST** exam: Face drooping, Arm weakness, Speech difficulty, Time to call help
- "Sudden onset" is key history since it suggests a vascular event. If so:
- Get stroke team NOW - don't try to figure out the type. IV access, check glucose
- An acute neurological change = potential stroke until proven otherwise.

### *Treatment of Stroke*

**Acute Management of Ischemic Stroke:**

In stroke, every minute counts. The door-to-needle time goal (the time from when the patient arrives at the hospital ["door"] to when tPA is administered ["needle"] is < 60 minutes for tPA. The door-to-groin time goal [the time from hospital arrival to when the catheter is inserted into the femoral artery ("groin") to begin the procedure] is < 90 minutes for thrombectomy.

- tPA (alteplase): Administer within 4.5 hours of symptom onset for eligible patients.
- Endovascular thrombectomy: May be performed up to 24 hours for large vessel occlusions IF advanced imaging shows salvageable brain tissue. The "time is brain" concept now includes tissue-based selection, not just time alone.
- In patients with acute ischemic stroke who are not receiving thrombolytic therapy (tPA): Blood pressure is usually not lowered unless it exceeds 220/120 mmHg (then keep <185/110). The rationale is to maintain adequate cerebral perfusion during the acute phase.
- In patients who are candidates for or are receiving intravenous tPA (alteplase): Blood pressure should be lowered to <185/110 mmHg before thrombolysis to reduce the risk of hemorrhagic transformation.
- Endovascular thrombectomy: May be performed up to 24 hours for large vessel occlusions IF advanced imaging shows salvageable brain tissue.

In a **transient ischemic attack (TIA)**, there is a brief interruption of blood flow in which the patient recovers, generally within 24 hours (most within 1 hour). While TIA is a risk for the development of a stroke (10-15% within 90 days if untreated), it does not have the same urgency and narrow window for action as a thrombotic stroke. The workup for a TIA is similar to that for an ischemic stroke, without the administration of tPA. Urgent workup includes vascular imaging and cardiac monitoring.

The risk for a future stroke following a TIA relates to its **ABCD$^2$** score (**A** = Age ≥60 yrs -> 1 point; **B** = Blood pressure ≥140/90 at presentation -> 1 point; **C** = Clinical features (e.g., weakness or speech disturbance) -> up to 2 points; **D** = Duration of symptoms -> up to 2 points; Diabetes -> 1 point).

TIAs are not candidates for tPA (by definition, symptoms have resolved).

- **Endovascular Thrombectomy:** May be indicated for patients with large artery occlusions in the anterior circulation within 24 hours of onset, who meet specific criteria, which take into account the size of the infarct, the degree of neurological deficit, and the medical stability of the patient.

**Secondary Prevention of Ischemic Stroke:**

- **Antiplatelets:** *Aspirin* initiated within 24-48 hours of stroke onset (not during tPA infusion); consider dual antiplatelet therapy with *clopidogrel* for more effective antiplatelet effect for the first 21-90 days in minor stroke/high-risk TIA.
- **Anticoagulation:** For patients with atrial fibrillation or other indications for systemic anticoagulation. Direct oral anticoagulants are preferred over warfarin for atrial fibrillation.
- **Statins:** High-intensity for atherosclerotic disease (e.g., *atorvastatin* 40–80 mg or *rosuvastatin* 20–40 mg)

**Risk Factor Management:** Control of hypertension, diabetes, dyslipidemia, and lifestyle modifications

The main treatment of cerebral venous thrombosis is anticoagulation (e.g., *heparin* followed by oral anticoagulants like *warfarin*). Increased intracranial pressure may need to be addressed with head elevation, osmotic diuretics (e.g., *mannitol*), or CSF fluid drainage. It is also important to address the underlying cause, whether an infective, inflammatory, or clotting disorder.

**Treatment of Hemorrhagic Stroke:**

**Blood Pressure Management:** Acute lowering of blood pressure is recommended to prevent hematoma expansion. Target a systolic BP of 140-179 mmHg. BP reduction in stroke must be gradual and carefully targeted, preserving perfusion to at-risk brain tissue. **Note:** For patients with acute *ischemic* stroke, lowering a high blood pressure may not be recommended, unless the BP is extremely high (e.g., > 220/120), as it might reduce needed perfusion to an already ischemic brain. Exact treatment guidelines may change.

**Surgical Intervention:** For patients with hemorrhage causing neurological deterioration and significant mass effect, or intraventricular hemorrhage with acute hydrocephalus, surgical evacuation or external ventricular drainage may be necessary.

**Reversal of Anticoagulation:** Specific reversal agents may be administered to an anticoagulated patient, depending on the anticoagulant the patient is on, whether it is a vitamin K antagonist (administer vitamin K), direct thrombin inhibitor, factor Xa inhibitor, *heparin* (administer *protamine sulfate* to reverse heparin effect), or other anticoagulant.

**Rehabilitation of Stroke:** Early initiation of rehabilitation interventions to address physical, cognitive, and speech impairments is important for maximizing recovery potential.

**A wake-up stroke** is a stroke of unknown onset time (about 25% of all strokes), discovered when a patient awakens, and may still be treatable based on brain imaging that shows viable tissue, although the patient may be ineligible for time-based interventions like tPA and thrombectomy.

Key messages:

- Time windows are longer than previously thought with proper patient selection.
- All stroke patients should go to comprehensive stroke centers when possible
- Don't assume it's "too late" - let the stroke team decide on treatment eligibility.
- Stroke mimics are common and affect treatment decisions.
- Secondary prevention is as important as acute treatment.

## Multiple Sclerosis

Multiple sclerosis (MS) is a chronic autoimmune disease that affects the central nervous system (CNS), leading to demyelination and neurodegeneration. It can have a wide range of neurological symptoms, since it can affect any area of the brain, brain stem, spinal cord, or optic nerves. The most common symptoms are:

- Muscle weakness or spasticity
- Fatigue
- Numbness or tingling, particularly of the limbs on one or both sides of the body
- Walking difficulties from weakness, spasticity, loss of balance, or sensory deficits
- Visual problems from optic neuritis, diplopia, or nystagmus
- Dizziness and vertigo
- Bladder or bowel dysfunction (urinary urgency, frequency, or retention; constipation or loss of bowel control); sexual dysfunction
- Cognitive changes, with problems of memory, attention, information processing, and executive function
- Mood swings, irritability, depression, or anxiety
- Pain, whether neuropathic (e.g., burning, stabbing, or sharp) or musculoskeletal
- Worsening of symptoms with increased body temperature
- *Lhermitte's sign*: A feeling of electric shock running down the back on neck flexion

Symptoms in most individuals manifest as periods of remission and relapse, but in some people, symptoms may evolve continuously.

*Diagnosis of Multiple Sclerosis (MS)*

The neurologist, in asking *where* the lesion is, tries to determine if a patient's cluster of symptoms and signs can all be explained by a single lesion. If it is necessary to postulate multiple lesions to account for the patient's findings, multiple sclerosis becomes a consideration, although there are other things that can also present as more than one lesion, e.g., metastatic disease; small vessel infarcts; certain infections; autoimmune, metabolic, and degenerative disorders; toxic and deficiency states; and the presence of more than one disease. The diagnosis of MS is based on the **McDonald criteria** (**Fig. 18-2**), which have been revised over the years. These criteria require the demonstration of disease dissemination in both time and space, with a focus on excluding other possible diagnoses.

Key components in the diagnostic process for MS include:

**Clinical Evaluation:** Assessment of historical and current symptoms suggestive of MS, along with a thorough neurological examination.

**Magnetic Resonance Imaging (MRI)** is the most sensitive non-invasive test for detecting MS plaques (lesions) in the CNS. MRI of the brain and spinal cord can show areas of demyelination, even if they're not causing symptoms. Gadolinium-enhancement of the MRI helps by highlighting the increased vascularity and leakage associated with inflammation.

**Cerebrospinal Fluid (CSF) Analysis:** While not required for all patients, CSF analysis can support the diagnosis by showing **oligoclonal bands** (distinct bands of immunoglobulins found in CSF but not in the serum) or **elevated IgG index** (the ratio of IgG to albumin in the CSF versus the ratio of IgG to albumin in the serum), which is indicative of an immune response within the CNS.

**FIGURE 18-2. THE MCDONALD CRITERIA FOR MULTIPLE SCLEROSIS**

***Dissemination in Space***

Lesions in at least two of four typical MS locations:

- Periventricular
- Cortical or juxtacortical (near the surface of the brain)
- Infratentorial (brain stem or cerebellum)
- Spinal cord

Alternatively: signs and symptoms indicating neurologic damage in at least two separate areas of the central nervous system

***Dissemination in Time (DIT)***

- The presence of gadolinium-enhancing lesions (indicating active inflammation) and non-enhancing lesions (indicating chronicity) at any time
- A new T2 or gadolinium-enhancing lesion on follow-up MRI, with the reference scan being at least 30 days after the onset of the initial clinical event. DIT can also be inferred if there is a new clinical attack implicating a different CNS site at a different time.

***Added Criteria***

- Symptomatic lesions in the optic nerve
- Oligoclonal bands (immunoglobulin bands indicating inflammation) in the CSF

**Evoked Potentials:** Measures the electrical activity of the brain in response to stimuli. The test can help identify demyelination along sensory pathways, even when symptoms are not present.

**Exclusion of Other Causes:** It's important to rule out other conditions that can mimic MS, including vitamin B12 deficiency (serum B12 levels); Lyme disease (serum or CSF Lyme disease antibodies; PCR of blood or CSF for *Borrelia burgdorferi* DNA); and various autoimmune disorders, such as lupus, Sjögren's syndrome, neuromyelitis optica spectrum disorder, and antiphospholipid syndrome (specific antibody tests).

***Treatment of Multiple Sclerosis***

Treatment of MS focuses on managing acute attacks, slowing disease progression, and addressing symptoms.

**Acute Relapses:** High-dose corticosteroids, typically intravenous *methylprednisolone*, are used to reduce inflammation and shorten the duration of relapses.

**Disease-Modifying Therapies (DMTs):** These drugs interact with the immune system and are aimed at reducing the frequency and severity of relapses, slowing the progression of disability, and limiting new disease activity as seen on MRI. There are several classes of DMTs, including injectables (e.g., *interferon beta, glatiramer acetate*), oral medications (e.g., *fingolimod, teriflunomide, dimethyl fumarate*), and monoclonal antibody infusions (e.g., *natalizumab, ocrelizumab, ofatumumab, alemtuzumab*). The choice of DMT depends on multiple factors, including disease activity, patient preference, side effect profile, and safety considerations. *Ponesimod* (*Ponvory*) is a selective sphingosine1phosphate (S1P) receptor modulator that limits lymphocyte migration into the central nervous system. *Briumvi* (*Ublitoximab*) is an antiCD20 monoclonal antibody that targets B cells, which are implicated in the autoimmune processes of MS.

**Symptomatic Treatment:** Addressing the various symptoms of MS (such as spasticity, fatigue, bladder and bowel dysfunction, pain, and cognitive issues) is essential for improving quality of life. This may involve pharmacological treatments, physical therapy, occupational therapy, and cognitive rehabilitation.

**Lifestyle Modifications and Support:** Regular exercise, a healthy diet, smoking cessation, and emotional support can help manage symptoms and improve overall well-being.

## Amyotrophic Lateral Sclerosis

Amyotrophic lateral sclerosis (ALS; Lou Gehrig's disease) is a progressive neurodegenerative disease that affects both upper and lower motor neurons in the brain and spinal cord. The loss of these neurons results in muscle weakness and atrophy, eventually leading to paralysis and death. On average, most individuals with ALS survive about two to five years after symptom onset, though some may live significantly longer.

### *Diagnosis of Amyotrophic Lateral Sclerosis*

**Physical examination** reveals an unusual aspect of ALS. ALS affects both upper *and* lower motor neurons, resulting in a mixture of upper and lower motor neuron signs. For instance, there may be atrophy and fasciculations of the hand muscles (lower motor neuron) combined with spasticity and hyperreflexia of the biceps and brachioradialis muscles (upper motor neuron). ALS may start off asymmetrically. Sensory loss is generally not a primary symptom. ALS often starts with muscle weakness in the hands, arms, legs, or muscles of speech and swallowing. It can eventually lead to breathing difficulties and death.

**Electromyography (EMG) and Nerve Conduction Studies (NCS)** measure the electrical activity of muscles and the speed and strength of nerve conduction, helping to identify signs of muscle or nerve dysfunction that may occur in ALS, and help to rule out other conditions.

**MRI** cannot diagnose ALS directly but can help rule out other conditions that might cause similar symptoms, such as spinal cord tumors or multiple sclerosis.

**Blood and Urine Tests:** These are used to exclude other diseases that may in some ways mimic ALS (e.g., thyroid disorders, electrolyte imbalances, kidney and liver disease, vitamin and mineral deficiencies, heavy metal poisoning, Lyme disease, HIV/AIDS, autoimmune diseases such as lupus or Sjögren's syndrome, and paraproteinemia (abnormally high levels of monoclonal antibody often found in multiple myeloma, Waldenstrom's macroglobulinemia, amyloidosis, and polyneuropathy).

**Spinal Tap** or **muscle biopsy** is sometimes done to rule out other nervous system diseases.

### *Treatment of Amyotrophic Lateral Sclerosis*

While there is presently no cure for ALS, treatments can help manage symptoms, prevent unnecessary complications, and make living with the disease as comfortable as possible. Treatment options include:

**Medications:**

- ***Riluzole (Rilutek)*** may slow the progression of ALS by its neuroprotective effect in inhibiting the release of glutamate from presynaptic neurons. Excess glutamate can be neurotoxic.

- *Edaravone (Radicava)* is an antioxidant drug that has been shown to slow the decline of physical function in ALS patients by neutralizing oxidative stress on neurons.
- **Relyvrio** (*sodium phenylbutyrate/taurursodiol*) is a combination therapy intended to help slow cellular processes (like mitochondrial dysfunction and endoplasmic reticulum stress) that contribute to motor neuron degeneration in ALS.

**Physical therapy** helps maintain mobility and manage symptoms.

**Occupational therapy** assists in finding ways to remain independent despite hand and arm weakness.

**Speech therapy** provides ways to maintain as much communication ability as possible, such as the use of alternative communication devices.

**Nutritional support** to help maintain weight and health

**Respiratory Therapy:** Ventilatory assistance might be necessary to aid breathing as the disease progresses.

**Psychological Support:** Counseling for patients and their families to cope with the emotional aspects of the disease

(new category above Cerebral Palsy with same font type) (italicize nusinersen):

***Spinal Muscular Atrophy***

Spinal Muscular Atrophy is a genetic neuromuscular disorder characterized by degeneration of the anterior horn cells (motor neurons) in the spinal cord, leading to progressive muscle weakness and atrophy, especially in proximal muscles. It is caused by a genetic mutation in the SMN1 gene. In infants, it can be fatal without treatment. Nusinersen, given by intrathecal injection, modifies how the SMN2 gene is spliced, leading to increased production of functional SMN protein, which is critical for motor neuron survival. It has transformed this disease from fatal to treatable.

## *Cerebral Palsy*

Cerebral palsy (CP) can have different symptomatic presentations, including problems with muscle stiffness, posture, contractures, balance and coordination, speech and swallowing, seizures, intellectual disability with developmental delay, vision and hearing, and emotional abnormalities. CP is caused by damage or abnormal development of the parts of the brain that control movement, balance, and posture. This damage can occur before, during, or shortly after birth, and the specific cause is not always identifiable. However, several risk factors and causes have been associated with the development of cerebral palsy:

**Prenatal Disturbances**: Genetic mutations, maternal infections (e.g., rubella, cytomegalovirus, toxoplasmosis), severe malnutrition, or exposure to toxins

**Premature Birth**: Premature babies, particularly those born before 32 weeks of gestation, have a higher risk of CP.

**Low Birth Weight**: Infants weighing less than 5.5 pounds at birth, and especially those weighing less than 3.3 pounds are at increased risk.

**Complicated labor and delivery** may lead to a lack of oxygen to the brain, severe jaundice, or head trauma.

**Multiple Births**: Twins, triplets, and other multiple births are at a higher risk.

**Blood Type Incompatibility**: Rh incompatibility leading to jaundice can cause brain damage.

**Infections in Infants**: Bacterial meningitis or viral encephalitis during infancy

**Stroke**: Perinatal strokes, which occur when blood flow to the brain is restricted or when there is bleeding in the brain around the time of birth

**Brain Injuries**: Brain damage resulting from accidents, falls, or child abuse during the first few years of life

*Diagnosis of Cerebral Palsy*

Cerebral palsy is diagnosed through history, physical exam, and often neuroimaging studies like MRI (sometimes CT or ultrasound) to look for abnormalities in brain structure. Genetic and metabolic testing, or EEG for seizures may also be helpful in diagnosis.

The child with cerebral palsy may present with:

**Muscle Tone Abnormalities**: This can range from spasticity to hypotonia. Spasticity is most common. **Motor milestone delays**, such as sitting up or crawling, can be early indicators of CP.

**Coordination and Balance Problems**: Difficulties with tasks that require fine motor skills, as well as problems with balance and walking, are common. This might include a wide gait or walking on toes (increased calf muscle tone).

**Involuntary Movements**: Uncontrolled, slow, writhing movements (athetosis) or rapid, jerky movements (chorea) can occur, especially in non-spastic forms of CP.

**Muscle Weakness and Paralysis**: Predominantly on one side of the body, but it can also affect both legs more than the arms (diplegia) or all four limbs (quadriplegia).

**Difficulty with Speech and Eating**: Issues with the muscles that control the mouth and throat can lead to difficulties with speech (dysarthria) and swallowing (dysphagia).

**Seizures**: A significant number of individuals with CP also have epilepsy, which can manifest as seizures.

**Cognitive Impairments**: While intelligence is unaffected in many people with CP, some may have intellectual disabilities.

**Sensory Impairments**: Vision, hearing, and tactile sensations may be affected.

**Orthopedic Problems**: Skeletal deformities, such as scoliosis, as well as joint problems, are common due to abnormal muscle tone and posture.

**Pain**: Chronic pain can result from spasticity, joint problems, or other complications.

**Developmental and Medical History**: Collecting detailed information about the child's prenatal, perinatal, and postnatal history, as well as the family's medical history, can provide clues to potential risk factors or causes of symptoms.

**Developmental Monitoring (Surveillance)**: This involves regularly tracking a child's growth and development to identify any delays or abnormalities in motor skills.

**Comprehensive Neurological Examination**: This examination focuses on identifying impairments in muscle tone, motor function, reflexes, and posture. The presence of abnormal muscle tone or reflexes can be indicative of CP.

**Neuroimaging**: Magnetic Resonance Imaging (MRI) is the preferred method for visualizing the brain's structure. It can identify abnormalities or injuries that may have contributed to CP. In some cases, cranial ultrasound (in infants) or computed tomography (CT) scans might also be used.

**Additional Tests**: Depending on the child's symptoms, other tests may include genetic testing, EEG for seizures, and testing for metabolic disorders that might mimic symptoms of CP. These include mitochondrial disorders (e.g., mitochondrial DNA depletion syndrome, myoclonic epilepsy with ragged red fibers), disorders of carbohydrate metabolism (e.g., glycogen storage diseases), acidemias (e.g., methylmalonic acidemia), urea cycle disorders (e.g., ornithine transcarbamylase deficiency), amino acidopathies (e.g., phenylketonuria; maple syrup urine disease), and disorders of fatty acid oxidation (e.g., carnitine deficiency).

*Treatment of Cerebral Palsy*

Treatment for CP is tailored to the individual's specific needs:

**Physical, Occupational and/or Speech and Language Therapy**

**Medication**: Muscle relaxants (e.g., *baclofen, diazepam*, or *botulinum toxin* injections) and pain relievers (e.g., NSAIDs) may be used to manage spasticity. Antiepileptic drugs may be prescribed for those with seizures.

**Orthopedic Interventions**: Surgical procedures may be necessary to correct skeletal deformities or to release tight muscles and tendons.

**Assistive Technology**: Devices such as braces, walkers, or wheelchairs can enhance mobility and independence.

**Nutritional Support**: A dietitian may be involved to address nutritional needs, especially if there are swallowing difficulties.

**Educational and Social Support**: Ensuring access to education and social activities is important for cognitive and social development.

## Peripheral Nervous System Causes of Weakness

These include peripheral neuropathies (discussed in **Chapter 20** – Numbness and Tingling), Guillain-Barré syndrome, Charcot-Marie-Tooth disease, and a variety of nerve injuries, such as carpal tunnel syndrome, ulnar and radial neuropathies, and direct trauma, e.g., from lacerations or fractures. Amyotrophic lateral sclerosis, which affects both the central and peripheral nervous system, is discussed above under Central Nervous System Causes of Weakness.

### Guillain-Barré Syndrome

Guillain-Barré Syndrome (GBS) is a rare neurological disorder in which the body's immune system mistakenly attacks the peripheral nervous system, both motor and sensory nerves. Symptoms include

weakness and tingling sensations, which can be painful, along with hyporeflexia. The symptoms usually start in the lower extremities and can symmetrically spread quickly, over hours or days, to the arms and upper body ("*ascending paralysis*"), with danger of paralysis and breathing difficulties in severe cases. Some people may have difficulty moving their eyes, speaking, chewing, or swallowing.

A spinal tap often shows increased protein without a significant increase in white blood cells (*albuminocytological dissociation*). Nerve conduction studies show slowed conduction velocities indicating demyelination or axon damage. EMG in later stages may show fibrillation and reduced muscle action potentials, indicating muscle denervation. Blood tests can look for signs of infections, which some believe may act as a trigger to cause GBS in some people.

Guillain-Barré is considered a medical emergency. Since it is an autoimmune disease, it is treated with intravenous immunoglobulins, or plasmapheresis to remove harmful immunoglobulins and immune complexes. Recovery may begin in about 2-4 weeks, but symptoms may last years.

## Neurologic Junction Causes Of Weakness

### *Myasthenia Gravis*

Myasthenia gravis (MG) is an autoimmune neuromuscular disorder characterized by the production of antibodies against the acetylcholine receptor (AChR), muscle-specific kinase (MuSK), or lipoprotein-related protein 4 (LRP4) at the neuromuscular junction, leading to muscle weakness and fatigue due to inadequate transmission of neural impulses to the muscles.

*Diagnosis of Myasthenia Gravis*

**Clinical Evaluation:** The hallmark is fluctuating muscle weakness, notably *improving with rest*. Ptosis, diplopia, and generalized weakness are common presenting symptoms.

**Lab Tests:** Antibodies against AChR are present in approximately 85% of generalized cases and 50% of ocular cases. Anti-MuSK or Anti-LRP4 antibodies may be found in cases negative for AChR antibodies.

**Electrophysiological Studies:**

- **Repetitive Nerve Stimulation (RNS)** shows a decreasing response in muscle action potential amplitude with repetitive stimulation.
- **Single Fiber Electromyography (SFEMG)** is considered the most sensitive test for MG, demonstrating increased *jitter* (the time it takes for one muscle fiber to follow the action potential of a neighboring fiber) and blocking (failure of neuromuscular transmission).

**Imaging:** Chest imaging, particularly CT or MRI, is important for thymoma detection. Thymomas are found in about 10-15% of patients with MG and may act as a trigger for the autoimmune response found in MG.

**Pharmacological Tests:** The *edrophonium* (*Tensilon*) test is less commonly used now due to its potential side effects (hypotension, arrhythmias, abdominal cramps, bronchospasm, headache, and dizziness). *Edrophonium*, given intravenously, can, through acetylcholinesterase inhibition, provide a rapid, though temporary (only about 5-10 minutes) improvement in strength in MG patients, helping to confirm the diagnosis. *Edrophonium* works by allowing more acetylcholine to be around to activate muscle contractions.

Treatment of Myasthenia Gravis

**Symptomatic Treatment:**

- **Cholinesterase Inhibitors:** *Pyridostigmine*, a cholinesterase inhibitor, is the mainstay for symptomatic treatment. Pyridostigmine has a longer duration of action, can be given orally, and has fewer side effects than edrophonium.

**Immunosuppression:**

- **Corticosteroids:** Prednisone is often used but needs careful management of side effects.

- **Steroid-sparing Agents:** *Azathioprine, mycophenolate mofetil,* and *cyclosporine* are options for long-term immunosuppression.
- **Intravenous immunoglobulin**: Infusion of normal antibodies (which may act in part by neutralizing autoantibodies or influencing the immune system in other ways) for short-term treatment of flare-ups
- **Rituximab**, a B-cell depleting monoclonal antibody, may be used in refractory cases or those with MuSK antibodies. Reducing the number of B cells decreases the production of the harmful autoantibodies in MG.
- ***Eculizumab***, a complement inhibitor, interferes with the damaging binding of complement to the neuromuscular junction in cases where there are antibodies against the acetylcholine receptors (AChR).
- ***Efgartigimod*** (***Vyvgart***) is an FcRn inhibitor that lowers levels of pathogenic IgG autoantibodies, thereby alleviating the autoimmune attack on neuromuscular junctions.
- **Plasmapheresis** or **Intravenous Immunoglobulin (IVIg):** Useful for exacerbations or preoperatively in thymectomy candidates. Both methods reduce circulating antibodies.

**Thymectomy:** Recommended for thymoma and considered for generalized MG without thymoma, as it can lead to remission or reduced medication needs.

### Botulism

Botulism is caused by the botulinum toxin, produced by the bacterium *Clostridium botulinum*. It commonly results from food poisoning or infected wounds. The symptoms may start with cranial nerve involvement (blurred vision, swallowing difficulties, muscle weakness) and progress as a descending paralysis, where the botulinum toxin prevents the release of acetylcholine at the neuromuscular junction. Botulism can be confirmed by mouse bioassay (injecting the suspected toxin into mice to observe for symptoms), serum analysis for botulinum toxin, or identification of *C. botulinum* in stool, or wound cultures. EMG and nerve conduction studies show decreased muscle response to stimulation.

Botulism is treated with early administration of botulinum antitoxin to neutralize the botulinum toxin in the bloodstream and prevent further damage. Mechanical ventilation, ICU monitoring, nutritional support, antibiotics for wound botulism, and elimination of contaminated food sources are all important measures. Antibiotics are not given for botulinum food poisoning since the poisoning arises from the botulinum toxin rather than an active bacterial infection. Honey should not be given to infants < 1yr old, who have a less mature immune system that cannot fight the *Clostridium botulinum* spores that may be in honey.

## Muscular Causes of Weakness

**Myopathies** are diseases that attack the muscles, leading to weakness, stiffness, or other muscle-related symptoms. They can affect skeletal and cardiac muscle, and sometimes smooth muscle (e.g., in the GI or urinary tract). Myopathies can be caused by genetic mutations, autoimmune reactions, infections, inflammation, or drug side effects.

## Muscular Dystrophy

The muscular dystrophies are a group of genetic myopathies with progressive muscle weakness and degeneration beginning in childhood or adolescence. They affect voluntary muscle movements like walking, running, lifting, and sometimes respiration. There is currently no cure. Treatment centers on managing symptoms and improving the quality of life with medication to slow the disease (e.g., corticosteroids, cardiac medication for cardiomyopathy; bronchodilators, mucolytics and antibiotics for respiratory involvement), physical therapy, assistive devices to help mobility (e.g., wheelchairs, scooters, walkers, canes), orthopedic interventions (braces, splints), and emerging therapies, such as gene and stem cell therapy.

*Eteplirsen* and *golodirsen* are drugs used to treat Duchenne muscular dystrophy (DMD) by promoting the production of functional dystrophin protein, which is deficient in DMD.

There are many kinds of muscular dystrophy. **Figure 18-3** lists the five most common forms. Diagnosis is based on clinical presentation, increased creatine kinase levels (a measure of muscle damage), genetic testing for gene mutations, and muscle biopsy.

## Polymyositis and Dermatomyositis

Polymyositis and dermatomyositis are autoimmune diseases where the body mistakenly attacks its own muscles, causing symmetrical, mainly proximal, muscle inflammation and weakness throughout the body. There may be a genetic component coupled with environmental triggers.

Dermatomyositis differs from polymyositis in exhibiting a distinctive skin rash, which may present as a heliotrope (purplish) discoloration around the eyes (**Fig. 18-4**), a scaly rash on the knuckles and extensor surfaces of the fingers (**Gottron's papules**) (**Fig. 18-5**), and a rash on areas exposed to the sun. Dermatomyositis also has a higher risk of malignancy than does polymyositis.

***Diagnosis of Polymyositis and Dermatomyositis***

**History and Physical Exam**: The patient may present with muscle weakness, fatigue, and (in dermatomyositis) skin changes.

**Lab Tests**:

- **Creatine Kinase (CK) Levels**: Elevated CK levels in blood tests may indicate muscle damage.
- **Autoantibody Testing**: Specific autoantibodies, such as anti-Jo-1 (polymyositis) or anti-Mi-2 (dermatomyositis), may be present. Anti-SRP antibodies may be found in other inflammatory myopathies (not discussed).
- **Inflammatory Markers**: Erythrocyte Sedimentation Rate (ESR) and C-reactive protein (CRP) may be elevated, indicating inflammation.

**Electromyography (EMG)**: EMG can help assess muscle function and detect abnormalities suggestive of myositis.

**Muscle Biopsy**: A muscle biopsy can confirm the diagnosis and assess the extent of muscle inflammation and damage.

**Imaging Studies**: MRI or ultrasound can detect muscle inflammation and characteristic patterns of muscle involvement.

| FIGURE 18-3. MUSCULAR DYSTROPHY | | |
|---|---|---|
| **Type of Muscular Dystrophy** | **Inheritance** | **Distinguishing Clinical Features** |
| **Duchenne Muscular Dystrophy (DMD)** | • X-linked recessive<br>• Defect in the gene for dystrophin, which is important for muscle function | • Mainly in boys<br>• Difficulty walking<br>• Delayed motor milestones<br>• Prominent calf enlargement<br>• Progressive disability<br>• Life expectancy may be extended into the 30s<br>• Treated with *eteplirsen* or *golodirsen* to help restore dystrophin |
| **Becker Muscular Dystrophy** | • X-linked recessive<br>• Defect in the gene for dystrophin, which is important for muscle function | • Mainly in boys<br>• Less severe than DMD, with longer life expectancy into 40s, 50s, or beyond |
| **Myotonic Dystrophy** | • Autosomal dominant<br>• Defect in the DMPK or CNBP gene | • Myotonia (delayed muscle relaxation after contraction)<br>• May lead to cardiac, pulmonary, and cognitive problems<br>• Life expectancy may be extended into the 50s, 60s, or longer<br>• Treated with anticonvulsants or *mexiletine* (blocks the overactive sodium channels in skeletal muscle fibers, thus reducing repetitive firing and easing muscle spasms and rigidity) to reduce myotonia and muscle stiffness |
| **Fascioscapulohumeral Muscular Dystrophy** | • Autosomal dominant<br>• Defect in the DUX4 gene | • Affects muscles of face, shoulders, and upper arms<br>• Often a normal life span |
| **Limb-Girdle Muscular Dystrophy** | • Autosomal dominant or recessive<br>• Defect in various genes affecting muscle function | • Affects muscles of shoulders and hips<br>• Often a normal life span |

*Treatment of Polymyositis and Dermatomyositis*

**Corticosteroids**: High-dose corticosteroids, such as *prednisone*, are typically the first-line treatment for polymyositis and dermatomyositis to suppress inflammation and reduce muscle weakness.

**Immunosuppressive Medications**: When corticosteroids alone are insufficient, immunosuppressive drugs such *as methotrexate, azathioprine, mycophenolate mofetil*, or *rituximab* may be added to control inflammation and reduce disease activity.

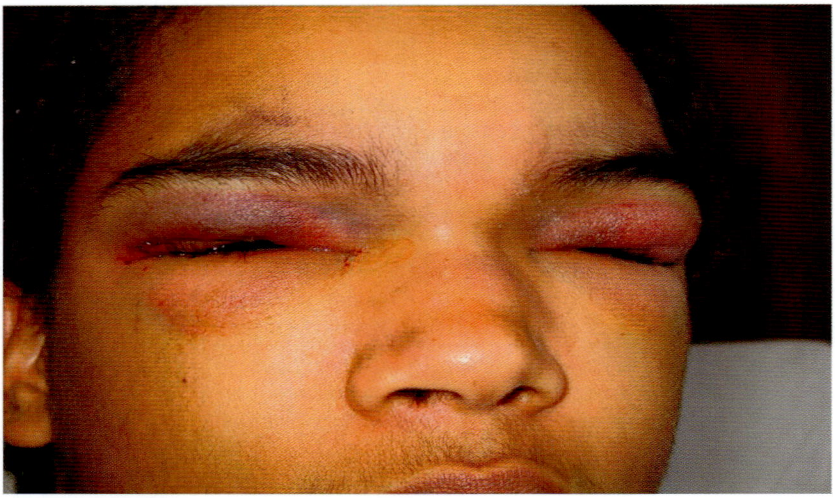

*Figure 18-4 Heliotrope rash in dermatomyositis.*

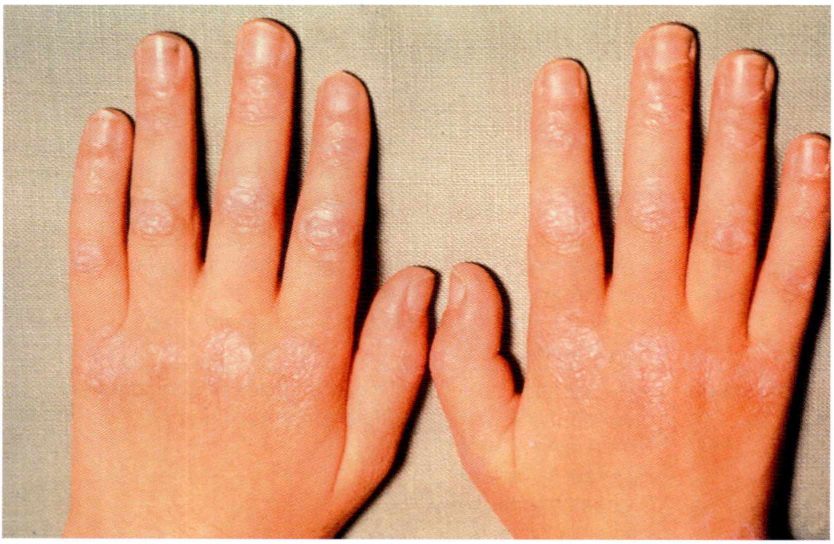

*Figure 18-5 Gottron's papules in dermatomyositis.*

**Physical Therapy**: Physical therapy can improve mobility, and prevent muscle atrophy.

**Skin Care**: For dermatomyositis, topical corticosteroids, moisturizers, and sun protection are important for managing skin symptoms.

**Supportive Care**: Symptomatic treatment may include pain management and psychological support to address the impact of the disease on the quality of life.

## *Statin Myopathy*

Statin myopathy is a potential side-effect of statins. The symptoms range from mild muscle aches to *rhabdomyolysis,* a severe condition with muscle breakdown, muscle pain and weakness. Muscle breakdown with release of myoglobin into the bloodstream can lead to kidney damage and electrolyte imbalance.

*Diagnosis of Statin Myopathy*

- Symptoms of muscle cramps, tenderness, or weakness should raise suspicion.
- Creatine kinase (CK) blood levels may be elevated, indicating muscle injury, although not all patients with statin myopathy have elevated CK.
- The urine may be tea-colored from the myoglobin.
- Other conditions should be ruled out, such as vitamin D deficiency, hypothyroidism, or physical overexertion, which can cause similar symptoms.
- Temporarily discontinuing the statin can be diagnostic if the symptoms disappear.

*Treatment of Statin Myopathy*

Treatment of statin myopathy consists of stopping the statin, reducing its dose, or switching to another statin or different cholesterol-lowering medication with less risk of myopathy.

Coenzyme Q10 supplements may help reduce the muscle symptoms, as can correction of a vitamin D deficiency. CoQ10 is a naturally occurring compound found in all cells of the body. It and vitamin D are important for muscle cell health. Statins can decrease CoQ10 levels.

# Metabolic Myopathies

Metabolic myopathies result from the inability of muscles to adequately metabolize energy. These myopathies include **glycogen storage diseases, fatty acid oxidation disorders**, and **mitochondrial myopathies**.

## *Glycogen Storage Diseases*

There are some 13 recognized glycogen storage diseases, all of which involve defects in the enzymes or proteins needed for glycogen synthesis and breakdown. This results in an abnormal accumulation or depletion of glycogen in the affected tissues, which may result in hepatomegaly, hypoglycemia, muscle weakness, and other systemic manifestations. Some of the better-known ones include:

**GSD Type I** (**von Gierke disease**): There is a deficiency in the enzyme *glucose-6-phosphatase*, leading to a decrease in the release of glucose from glycogen. Glycogen accumulates in the liver and kidneys, along with hypoglycemia.

**GSD Type II** (**Pompe disease**): There is a deficiency in the enzyme *alpha-glucosidase*, which is needed for breaking down glycogen into glucose in lysosomes. Glycogen accumulates in the lysosomes, causing progressive muscle weakness. There may be dizziness, syncope, or arrhythmias.

**GSD Type III** (**Cori disease**): There is a deficiency in the *glycogen debranching enzyme,* which is needed for glycogen breakdown. Abnormal glycogen accumulates, resulting in hepatomegaly and hypoglycemia. There may also be peripheral neuropathy, ataxia, tremor, or cognitive impairment.

**GSD Type IV (Andersen disease)**: There is a mutation in the *glycogen branching enzyme*, leading to the accumulation of abnormal glycogen structures, with hepatomegaly, liver dysfunction, and hypoglycemia. There may also be developmental delay, intellectual disability, hypotonia, seizures, skeletal muscle weakness, respiratory dysfunction, and cardiomyopathy.

**GSD Type V (McArdle disease)**: There is a deficiency in the enzyme *muscle glycogen phosphorylase*, which is important in the breakdown of muscle glycogen. There is an inability to break down glycogen to glucose during exercise, resulting in exercise intolerance, muscle cramps, and myoglobinuria.

**Diagnosis of glycogen storage diseases** involves a thorough medical history and physical examination, which may show signs and symptoms of GSD, such as hepatomegaly, hypoglycemia, growth retardation, muscle weakness, and exercise intolerance. Blood tests can assess glucose levels, liver enzymes, and markers of muscle damage, including elevated levels of creatine kinase, aldolase, myoglobin, LDH, AST, and ALT (LDH, AST, and ALT are found in muscle as well as liver and other tissues).

**Genetic testing** can identify mutations in genes associated with specific types of GSD, confirming the diagnosis and guiding treatment decisions. This testing may involve DNA sequencing or other molecular techniques.

**Imaging studies** like ultrasound, MRI, or CT scans may be used to evaluate the size and appearance of the liver and other affected organs.

The **treatment of glycogen storage diseases** involves dietary modifications. The aim is to maintain normal blood glucose levels, control hyperlipidemia (lipids may be called upon for energy when glucose is not available), and reduce liver size and fibrosis (e.g., with lipid-lowering drugs). In the case of Pompe disease, enzyme replacement with *alpha-glucosidase* is available. Liver transplantation may be considered for severe cases of GSD.

## Fatty Acid Oxidation Disorders

Fatty acid oxidation disorders (FAODs) are a group of rare inherited metabolic disorders characterized by defects in the enzymes responsible for breaking down fatty acids for energy. This results in muscle weakness, among other symptoms.

### *Diagnosis of Fatty Acid Oxidation Disorders*

The diagnosis of FAODs typically involves several steps:

**History:** FAODs often present with symptoms such as hypoglycemia (low blood sugar), lethargy, poor feeding, failure to thrive, muscle weakness, and liver dysfunction. Given the nonspecific nature of these symptoms, diagnosis may require a high index of suspicion, particularly in cases with a family history of FAODs or suggestive clinical features.

**Lab Tests:** Blood tests can assess levels of specific fatty acids, elevated acylcarnitines (intermediate metabolites of fatty acid oxidation), and organic acids (elevated ketones and dicarboxylic acids due to impaired breakdown of fatty acids for energy). There may be hypoglycemia due to the reliance on glucose metabolism for energy production rather than fatty acid oxidation. Genetic testing may also be performed to identify mutations in genes associated with FAODs.

**Imaging studies**, such as MRI may be used to evaluate for structural abnormalities in the liver, heart, and other organs, which can occur in some types of FAODs.

**Confirmatory Testing**: Definitive diagnosis of FAODs often requires confirmatory testing, such as enzyme activity assays or molecular genetic testing to identify specific enzyme deficiencies or genetic mutations associated with the disorder.

*Treatment of Fatty Acid Oxidation Disorders*

**Dietary Management**: The mainstay of treatment for FAODs involves dietary modifications to minimize the accumulation of toxic metabolites and provide alternative energy sources. This often includes a low-fat, high-carbohydrate diet, frequent meals/snacks, and avoidance of fasting.

**Medical Management**: Some individuals with FAODs may benefit from supplementation with medium-chain triglycerides (MCT oil), carnitine, or riboflavin to help bypass defective enzyme pathways or support fatty acid metabolism. Apart from supplements, symptomatic treatment of complications such as hypoglycemia or metabolic acidosis (from accumulation of organic acids and ketone bodies) may be necessary during acute episodes.

**Avoidance of Triggers**: Certain triggers such as prolonged fasting, illness, or high-fat meals can exacerbate symptoms in individuals with FAODs. Avoidance of these triggers is essential to prevent metabolic decompensation.

**Lifestyle Modifications**: Regular monitoring of growth, development, and metabolic parameters is important for individuals with FAODs.

## Mitochondrial Myopathies

Mitochondrial myopathies are a group of rare genetic disorders that result from defects in mitochondrial DNA or nuclear DNA encoding proteins essential for mitochondrial function. Those that originate in mitochondrial DNA are maternally inherited. Those originating in nuclear DNA can be autosomal dominant, autosomal recessive, X-linked, or sporadic. Symptoms can appear at any age, from infancy to adulthood, depending on the myopathy. Since mitochondria are essential for energy production, there can be a wide range of symptoms affecting multiple organ systems. Some of the more common mitochondrial myopathies include:

- MELAS (Mitochondrial Encephalomyopathy, Lactic Acidosis, and Stroke-like Episodes)
- MERRF (Myoclonic Epilepsy with Ragged Red Fibers)
- LS (Leigh Syndrome)
- CPEO (Chronic Progressive External Ophthalmoplegia)
- MNGIE (Mitochondrial Neurogastrointestinal Encephalopathy)
- LHON (Leber's Hereditary Optic Neuropathy)
- MDDS (Mitochondrial DNA Depletion Syndromes)

Neurological symptoms that may occur in all the mitochondrial myopathies include muscle weakness, exercise intolerance, muscle cramps, peripheral neuropathy, ataxia, myoclonus (brief, involuntary muscle jerks), seizures (especially with MELAS or MERRF), cognitive impairment, stroke-like episodes (especially with MELAS), optic neuropathy (especially with LHON), and hearing loss. Other problems include cardiomyopathy and gastrointestinal symptoms, e.g., dysphagia, GI dysmotility, abdominal pain, vomiting, and diarrhea. There may also be respiratory insufficiency, endocrine dysfunction, renal impairment, and developmental delays.

*Diagnosis of Mitochondrial Myopathies*
**Blood Tests**:

- Serum lactate and pyruvate are elevated, since mitochondrial ATP synthesis is interrupted, with a shift to anaerobic glycolysis, where lactate and pyruvate are produced.
- Elevated creatine kinase reflects muscle damage.
- CBC, electrolytes, liver and renal function tests, thyroid function tests, and metabolic panels can identify systemic abnormalities.

**Muscle biopsy** can identify the specific myopathy.
**Imaging studies** (MRI, CT) can detect signs of muscle pathology.
**Genetic testing** can identify specific mutations in mitochondrial or nuclear DNA.
**EMG and nerve conduction studies** can assess peripheral nerve and muscle function.

***Treatment of mitochondrial myopathies*** partly focuses on managing symptoms, such as muscle weakness and pain. Physical and occupational therapy can help improve daily functioning. Coenzyme Q10 enhances ATP production and may be used to improve mitochondrial function. Dietary supplements, apart from vitamins and minerals, may include *carnitine* (an important component of mitochondrial energy metabolism), *creatine* (enhances ATP regeneration), and antioxidants (reduces oxidative stress) to improve mitochondrial function. It is important for the patient to try to avoid any triggers that might exacerbate the symptoms, such as extreme temperatures, infections, and certain medications, e.g., statins, tetracyclines, aminoglycosides, some chemotherapy drugs, *valproic acid* (an antiepileptic), and certain anesthetics, all of which have been associated with mitochondrial toxicity. Systemic issues such as cardiac and respiratory problems and neurologic symptoms should be addressed. Current experimental therapies are being investigated.

## Periodic Paralysis

Periodic paralysis refers to a group of rare genetic muscle disorders characterized by episodes of muscle weakness or paralysis that occur intermittently. The two main types of periodic paralysis are **hypokalemic periodic paralysis (HPP)** and **hyperkalemic periodic paralysis (HYPP).** Hypokalemia *decreases* the excitability of muscle cells, and nerves cannot efficiently transmit signals to the muscle cells. Hyperkalemia *increases* excitability of the muscle cells, with easier muscle fatigue and weakness.

*Diagnosis of Periodic Paralysis*

**History and Physical Exam**: There may be a family history and triggers associated with episodes of weakness or paralysis. The exam may reveal muscle weakness and hypotonia (less resistance to passive movement), with diminished reflexes.

**Serum Potassium Levels**: In hypokalemic periodic paralysis (HPP), episodes of weakness are typically associated with low serum potassium levels during attacks, whereas in hyperkalemic periodic paralysis (HYPP), serum potassium levels are elevated during attacks.

**Thyroid Function Tests**: Thyroid function should be evaluated, as certain thyroid disorders can mimic symptoms of periodic paralysis.

**Genetic Testing**: Genetic testing can confirm the diagnosis and identify mutations in genes associated with periodic paralysis.

**Electromyography (EMG)**: EMG can help assess muscle function and detect abnormalities in nerve-muscle communication during episodes of weakness.

**Provocative Testing**: Provocative tests, such as oral potassium or glucose tolerance tests (glucose may trigger an attack of periodic paralysis in some people), may be performed to induce and characterize episodes of weakness and assess response to treatment.

*Treatment of Periodic Paralysis*

**Hypokalemic Periodic Paralysis (HPP)**: During attacks of weakness, oral or intravenous potassium supplementation can help restore serum potassium levels and alleviate symptoms.

**Hyperkalemic Periodic Paralysis (HYPP)**: During attacks, oral glucose administration (glucose drives potassium into cells), or intravenous administration of glucose and insulin, may be used to alleviate symptoms.

**Dietary Modifications**: Patients with periodic paralysis may benefit from dietary modifications to help prevent episodes, such as avoiding triggers like high-carbohydrate meals or fasting in HPP, and avoiding potassium-rich foods in HYPP.

**Medications**: Certain medications, such as *acetazolamide* or *dichlorphenamide* (carbonic anhydrase inhibitors, which can lower serum potassium levels), may be used as prophylactic treatment to reduce the frequency and severity of attacks in some cases of periodic paralysis.

**Lifestyle Modifications**: Lifestyle measures (such as maintaining adequate hydration, avoiding extreme temperatures, managing stress, and getting regular exercise) may help minimize the frequency and severity of attacks.

**Genetic Counseling**: Genetic counseling is recommended for individuals with periodic paralysis and their families to discuss the genetic inheritance pattern (which can be autosomal dominant or autosomal recessive), the risk of passing the condition to offspring, and available testing and treatment options.

# 19

# *Dizziness and Vertigo*

**Vertigo** is a sensation of spinning or movement, either of the self or the environment. **Dizziness** is a lightheaded, faint feeling without a sense of spinning. Vertigo is due to a dysfunction of the vestibular system, whether in the periphery (e.g., benign paroxysmal positional vertigo, Ménière's disease, vestibular neuritis, labyrinthitis) or a problem in the brain, like stroke or tumor (**Fig. 19-1**).

*Diagnostic Approach to Dizziness and Vertigo*

**Clinical History**

It is important to determine if vertigo is of central or peripheral origin. Collect information about the onset, duration, frequency, and triggers of episodes, associated symptoms such as hearing loss or tinnitus (suggesting a peripheral cause) or neurologic symptoms like weakness or dysarthria (suggesting a central cause). Dizziness may be triggered by standing up quickly (in orthostatic hypotension). Vertigo, frequently accompanied by nausea and vomiting, balance problems, difficulty walking, and nystagmus, and sometimes hearing changes, is often triggered by changes in head position, a peripheral cause.

3 Main Questions:

QUESTION 1: "Are you dizzy or is the room spinning?"

- Dizzy / lightheaded = Blood pressure, heart, anxiety
- Room spinning (vertigo) = Ear or brain problem

| FIGURE 19-1. CAUSES OF DIZZINESS AND VERTIGO |
|---|
| **INNER EAR PROBLEMS**<br>**Benign Paroxysmal Positional Vertigo (BPPV):** Tiny calcium particles clump up in the canals of the inner ear, causing brief episodes of vertigo.<br>**Ménière's Disease:** A chronic ("many years disease") intermittent inner ear disorder manifest as episodes of vertigo, tinnitus, and hearing loss<br>**Vestibular Neuritis:** Infection (commonly thought to be viral) or inflammation of the inner ear causes dizziness and balance issues. Vertigo typically starts suddenly, the acute phase lasting continuously about a week, generally without hearing loss or tinnitus.<br>**Labyrinthitis:** Affects the vestibular apparatus, like vestibular neuritis, but also the cochlea, causing hearing loss, too<br>**Acoustic Neuroma** |
| **INFECTIONS**<br>**Viral infections** of the inner ear or brain.<br>**Bacterial infections**, including middle ear infections or meningitis. |
| **NEUROLOGICAL DISORDERS**<br>**Migraine:** Some people experience dizziness or vertigo as part of their migraine episodes.<br>**Stroke:** Sudden dizziness or vertigo, trouble walking, or loss of balance could indicate a stroke.<br>**Multiple Sclerosis (MS):** Can cause dizziness or vertigo due to nerve damage and demyelination |
| **CARDIOVASCULAR CAUSES OF DIZZINESS OR VERTIGO**<br>**Arrhythmia**<br>**Orthostatic hypotension, cardiomyopathy, heart attack, and other heart conditions** that affect circulation |
| **MEDICATIONS**<br>**Side effects of medications** can include dizziness or vertigo, especially those that affect blood pressure or the central nervous system. |
| **HEAD INJURY**<br>**Concussion** (a mild traumatic brain injury without structural damage) can lead to symptoms of headache, dizziness or vertigo, and cognitive impairment. |
| **PSYCHOLOGICAL FACTORS**<br>**Anxiety Disorders:** Panic attacks and anxiety can cause episodes of dizziness or vertigo.<br>**Depression:** Sometimes associated with dizziness or vertigo |
| **OITHER CAUSES OF DIZZINESS OR VERTIGO**<br>**Dehydration or heatstroke**<br>**Hypoglycemia**<br>**Anemia**<br>**Age-related decline in ear function**<br>**Excess alcohol consumption or substance use**<br>**Vision problems**<br>**Cervical Spine Disorders:** Through proprioceptive dysfunction, vertebral artery compression, or muscular trigger point tension that can affect circulation or nerve signals |

QUESTION 2: "When does it happen?"
- When standing up = Orthostatic hypotension (check BP lying/standing)
- With head movement = Benign paroxysmal positional vertigo (BPPV)
- All the time = More concerning (brain, medication)

QUESTION 3: "Any hearing changes?"
- Yes = Ear problem (Meniere's, infection)
- No = Could be brain stem or BPPV

Dizziness Red Flags:
- New neurologic symptoms (weakness, numbness)
- Sudden severe dizziness
- Hearing loss
- Can't walk due to dizziness

Simple Rule: Vertigo + neurologic symptoms = brain problem (emergency)

**Physical Exam for Vertigo**

**Head Impulse Test (HIT):** The normal vestibulo-ocular reflex stabilizes vision by producing eye movements in the opposite direction of head movement, thus keeping vision fixated on a target. Look for vestibulo-ocular reflex failure on rapidly turning the patient's head to either side, suggesting a peripheral cause.

**Observation for Nystagmus:** Nystagmus of peripheral origin shows fatigability, i.e., the nystagmus tends to decrease with continuous exposure to the triggering position. Central nystagmus generally is not fatigable and persists despite the frequency or duration of the position that induces it.

**Romberg Test** (described in **Chapter 12** – The Neurologic Exam) and **Fukuda Stepping Test** (the patient is asked to march with the eyes closed) to assess for balance and vestibular function. Failure to keep balance in these tests suggests a problem with vestibular function if proprioception is normal.

In the **Dix-Hallpike maneuver** (rapidly moving the patient from a sitting to a supine position with the head turned to one side and hanging slightly over the edge of the table), nystagmus and vertigo suggest benign positional vertigo. In the **Roll test** (the patient lies flat and then the head is quickly turned to one side and then the other, vertigo and nystagmus suggest *canalithiasis* (calcium carbonate crystals [*otoconia*] displaced into the semicircular canals) as a cause for benign paroxysmal positional vertigo.

**Imaging and Additional Testing:**

**MRI** of the brain is important in evaluating for central causes of vertigo, such as stroke or multiple sclerosis, particularly if there are any other neurologic signs or symptoms. MRI or CT scan may also detect an acoustic neuroma or other abnormalities of inner ear anatomy.

**Audiometric tests** (for hearing loss patterns: E.g., Ménière's disease typically shows hearing loss in the low- to mid-frequency range, whereas labyrinthitis often shows hearing loss in the high frequency range. Hearing loss is usually not affected in vestibular neuritis.

**Vestibular function tests** can help identify peripheral disorders, such as Ménière's disease or vestibular neuritis. E.g., *videonystagmography* precisely measures eye movements

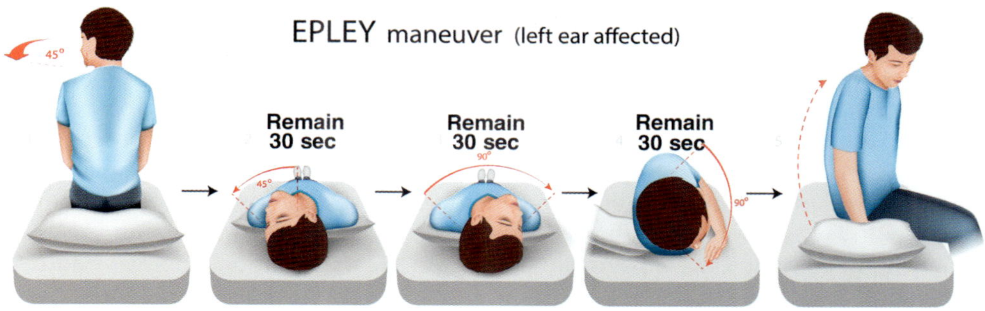


*Figure 19-2 The Epley maneuver for benign positional vertigo. The affected ear is the one turned down during the period of most intense vertigo.*

on camera. *Electronystagmography* measures eye movements with electrodes placed around the eyes.

*Treatment of Vertigo*

Distinguishing between peripheral and central vertigo guides treatment. Peripheral causes are more common and often have a more benign course.

**Peripheral Vertigo:**

- **Benign Paroxysmal Positional Vertigo:** The **Epley maneuver** (**Fig. 19 -2**) is effective in treating BPPV by repositioning canaliths within the inner ear. It may have to be repeated several times to be effective.
- **Vestibular Neuritis:** Corticosteroids can reduce inflammation. Vestibular rehabilitation exercises, guided by a physical or occupational therapist trained in vestibular rehabilitation therapy, help recovery. For labyrinthitis, antibiotics may be used if a bacterial infection is suspected.
- **Ménière's Disease:** Treatment includes dietary salt restriction, diuretics (as Ménière's may relate to abnormal fluid volumes in the inner ear), and in severe cases, administration behind the eardrum of *gentamicin* (for its ototoxic effects in decreasing the sensitivity of the vestibular system) or, in refractory cases, surgical options (e.g., vestibular nerve section).

**Central Vertigo:** Management focuses on treating the underlying cause, such as stroke or multiple sclerosis. Vestibular rehabilitation (gaze stabilization exercises, balance and gait training) may also be helpful for symptom relief in central vertigo. This can involve retraining the brain to recognize and process signals from the vestibular system more effectively, head and body movement exercises, eye exercises to improve visual stability, and balance training, generally conducted by a trained physical therapist or audiologist.

**Symptomatic Management**

**Medications:** For infections, antibiotics may help. Antihistamines (such as *meclizine*), benzodiazepines (for acute episodes), and antiemetics can be used for symptomatic relief of nausea and motion sickness. Long-term use of vestibular suppressants is generally discouraged, to allow the brain time to adapt naturally.

### *Treatment of Dizziness Without Vertigo*

Treatment of dizziness without vertigo depends on the cause. Increased fluid and salt intake to raise blood volume will help if the cause is dehydration and low blood volume. Gradual changes in posture on arising, compression stockings, and increased salt and water intake, or medications to increase blood pressure (e.g., *fludrocortisone; midodrine; pyridostigmine*) can help orthostatic hypotension. If the dizziness is due to medication or medication side effect, changing the medication or altering its dosage may help. Psychotherapy (e.g., cognitive-behavioral therapy), relaxation techniques, and medication may help manage symptoms of psychological origin. Heart conditions should be addressed.

# 20

# *Numbness and Tingling*

Numbness and tingling (*paresthesias*) can occur anywhere in the body but are most reported in the hands, arms, legs, and feet. They can be chronic or transient, mild or severe, and arise from a problem in the central or peripheral nervous system. Localizing the lesion is an important first step.

Transient paresthesias often result from nerve compression, such as falling asleep on an arm or leg, but can also be chronic, the result of peripheral neuropathy (e.g., diabetes or vitamin deficiency), multiple sclerosis, carpal tunnel syndrome, radiculopathy (symptoms from nerve *root* compression), or circulatory conditions (**Fig. 20-1**). Underlying all these is damage or excess stimulation of peripheral nerve fiber communication with the brain.

### *Diagnosis of Numbness and Tingling*

**History**

- *When did the symptoms begin and how did they progress?* Sudden onset suggests an acute injury. Gradual onset may suggest a chronic condition such as a neuropathy or systemic disease. Intermittent symptoms may suggest conditions that have flare-ups or remissions, e.g., multiple sclerosis, migraines, complex regional pain syndrome, *neuromyelitis optica* (*Devic's disease* – a chronic CNS disorder with inflammation and demyelination of the optic nerves and spinal cord), lupus, or episodic peripheral neuropathies (sometimes familial).
- *Are the paresthesias localized or generalized?* Strictly localized paresthesia suggests a localized nerve injury (e.g., carpal tunnel syndrome, ulnar neuropathy). A dermatomal distribution suggests nerve root compression, as in a radiculopathy. In carpal tunnel syndrome paresthesias are felt in the median nerve distribution, in the thumb, index finger, middle finger and thumb side of the ring finger. In ulnar neuropathy they are

**FIGURE 20-1. CAUSES OF NUMBNESS AND TINGLING (PARESTHESIAS)**

**Neurological Causes of Numbness and Tingling**

- Peripheral Neuropathy
- Cervical Spondylosis (may cause nerve root compression, inflammation, or decreased blood flow)
- Stroke or TIA
- Multiple Sclerosis
- Guillain-Barré Syndrome
- Complex Regional Pain Syndrome (caused by injury to a limb, e.g., fracture or surgery)
- Restless Legs Syndrome

**Vascular Causes of Numbness and Tingling**

- Raynaud's Phenomenon (due to constriction of blood vessels in the extremities)
- Peripheral Artery Disease (ischemia)

**Metabolic and Endocrine Causes of Numbness and Tingling**

- Diabetes (damages small blood vessels supplying nerves)
- Hypothyroidism (altered metabolism; possible nerve compression from myxedema)
- Vitamin B12 Deficiency (defects in the myelin sheath, deterioration of spinal cord white matter pathways carrying touch)
- Electrolyte Imbalances (hypocalcemia, hypo- or hyperkalemia, hypomagnesemia, hyponatremia)
- Renal Failure (uremia, electrolyte imbalances, acid-base disorders)
- Amyloid Neuropathy (accumulation of amyloid proteins can affect peripheral nerves)

**Infectious Causes of Numbness and Tingling**

- Lyme Disease (caused by a tick bite with Borrelia bacterium. The patient may have fever, headache, fatigue, *erythema migrans* skin rash, and peripheral neuropathy if not treated with antibiotics.
- HIV/AIDS (HIV virus can directly damage nerve fibers or make them susceptible to other infections)
- Herpes Zoster (shingles)

**Toxins and Medications Causing Numbness and Tingling**

- Heavy Metal Poisoning
- Certain Medications (chemotherapy, antiretroviral drugs, etc.)

**Lifestyle Factors Causing Numbness and Tingling**

- Alcohol Abuse (can lead to peripheral neuropathy)
- Repetitive Stress Injuries

**Immune Diseases Causing Numbness and Tingling**

- Lupus (inflammation and damage to peripheral nerves or blood vessels)
- Rheumatoid Arthritis (inflammation can affect nerves)
- Sarcoidosis (inflammatory granulomas can affect any area of the nervous system)
- Sjögren's Syndrome (autoimmune attack and inflammation causing peripheral neuropathy; autonomic neuropathy, including dry eyes and mouth; cognitive difficulties; and mood changes)
- Multiple Myeloma (from nerve compression, amyloidosis, chemotherapy side effects, or immunoglobulin M (IgM) deposits from the cancerous plasma cells)
- Waldenstrom's macroglobulinema (excess immunoglobulin M from abnormal B cells can affect nerves)
- POEMS syndrome (**P**olyneuropathy, **O**rganomegaly, **E**ndocrinopathy, **M**onoclonal protein, **S**kin changes)(Abnormal growth of plasma cells produces abnormal proteins that can damage peripheral nerves.)
- Light chain amyloidosis (amyloid can deposit in nerves)
- Paraneoplastic syndromes (arise from the body's response to substances produced by a tumor)

**Temporary Causes of Numbness and Tingling**

- Pressure on a nerve (carpal tunnel syndrome, cubital tunnel syndrome, thoracic outlet syndrome, herniated disc, tarsal tunnel syndrome, piriformis syndrome)
- Hyperventilation (reduced CO2 levels can cause blood vessel constriction and decreased nerve function)

**Idiopathic**

felt in the ulnar distribution to the little finger, inner half of the ring finger and part of the palm and back of the hand (**Fig. 10-2**). Glove-and-stocking paresthesia suggests a peripheral neuropathy, while a band-like sensation around the torso may suggest a spinal cord thoracic lesion.

- *Are the paresthesias unilateral or bilateral?* Unilateral paresthesias can indicate focal trauma or infection. Bilateral symptoms are more suggestive of a generalized neuropathy (e.g., diabetic neuropathy, metabolic disorders, toxic exposures, or widespread inflammation (e.g., Guillain-Barré syndrome).
- *Are there any other accompanying symptoms,* e.g., weakness, pain, changes in bowel or bladder function, or alterations in coordination or gait? This information aids in localizing the problem. Changes in bowel or bladder function may suggest a spinal cord lesion or multiple sclerosis. A problem with coordination raises the possibility of cerebellar involvement.
- *Does anything exacerbate or relieve the symptoms?* For instance, cold or emotional stress can evoke narrowing of blood vessels and compromise of blood flow to nerves in **Raynaud's phenomenon**. A peripheral neuropathy may worsen at night and improve with walking. Symptoms due to spinal stenosis may worsen on walking. If splinting helps, splinting might be considered as a treatment modality.
- *Is there a history of chronic illness,* e.g., diabetes or thyroid disorders?

**Neurologic Exam**

**Sensory Exam**: The nature of any sensory deficits can provide diagnostic clues. *Diabetic neuropathy* commonly presents in a glove-and-stocking distribution. *Radiculopathies* from nerve root irritation often present in a dermatome distribution. Disorders of the nerve plexuses, e.g., *brachial plexus injury*, present with sensory deficits in the plexus distribution (**Fig. 10-2**). Mononeuropathies, e.g., *carpal tunnel syndrome* (median nerve) or *meralgia paresthetica* (lateral femoral cutaneous nerve), lead to deficits in specific nerve territories. *Multiple sclerosis* can present with patchy defects, *stroke* with contralateral defects, *spinal cord lesions* with bilateral deficits below the level of the lesion.

**Motor Exam**: A combination of motor and sensory deficits that conform to a single nerve distribution, suggests a peripheral lesion; if it doesn't conform to a single nerve distribution, there may be a central lesion. Conditions affecting muscles typically present with muscle weakness without sensory disturbances, while conditions affecting nerves may affect both motor and sensory function. Muscle atrophy, fasciculations, and hyporeflexia suggest a lower motor neuron lesion. Hyperreflexia without significant atrophy or fasciculations suggests an upper motor lesion.

**Blood Tests**: Comprehensive metabolic panel, vitamin B12 levels, thyroid function tests, and glucose levels to rule out metabolic causes

**Electrodiagnostic Studies**: Nerve conduction studies (NCS) and electromyography (EMG) to evaluate the integrity and function of peripheral nerves and muscles

**Imaging**: MRI of the brain or spinal cord may be indicated if a central cause is suspected, such as multiple sclerosis or spinal cord compression.

**Lumbar Puncture**: Considered if there is suspicion of central nervous system involvement, to analyze cerebrospinal fluid for inflammatory or infectious conditions

**Other Tests**: Depending on the clinical context, tests for specific conditions, such as autoimmune disorders and infectious diseases, or genetic testing for hereditary neuropathies, may be warranted.

## Peripheral Neuropathy

Peripheral neuropathy refers to a range of conditions characterized by damage to the peripheral nervous system. This impairs the proper transmission of signals, resulting in symptoms that can include weakness, numbness, tingling, pain, and altered function in the affected areas. The onset of a peripheral neuropathy can be acute or chronic, and the progression can be steady or episodic.

Peripheral neuropathies can be classified in several ways:

A. *Classification Based on the **Number** of Nerves Involved.* **Mononeuropathies** involve damage to a single peripheral nerve (e.g., carpal tunnel syndrome or ulnar nerve palsy). **Multiple mononeuropathies (Mononeuritis Multiplex)** involve two or more nerves in different body areas (e.g., vasculitis, diabetes). **Polyneuropathies** involve many peripheral nerves throughout the body (e.g. diabetic polyneuropathy).

B. *Classification Based on the **Type** of Nerve Involved.* **Motor nerve neuropathies** *cause problems with movement.* **Sensory nerve neuropathies** *affect sensation; the patient may experience tingling, numbness, or pain.* **Autonomic neuropathies** *involve autonomic nerves and may affect blood pressure, heart rate, digestion, and bladder function.* **Sensorimotor neuropathies** *affect both motor and sensory nerves, causing motor and sensory problems.*

C. *Classification Based on the **Pattern** of Nerve Involvement.* **Distal symmetric polyneuropathies** *affect both sides of the body, particularly the nerves that extend most distally, e.g., to the feet.* **Asymmetric polyneuropathies** *affect different nerves in different places.*

D. *Classification Based on the **Underlying Cause**:*
   - Diabetic neuropathy
   - Toxic neuropathy (e.g., from chemotherapy or heavy metals)
   - Hereditary neuropathies, e.g., **Charcot-Marie-Tooth**, a sensorimotor neuropathy (commonly autosomal dominant or autosomal recessive) with muscle weakness, atrophy, decreased reflexes, and sensory loss, mainly in the feet and legs, later in the hands and arms. There often are foot deformities.
   - Inflammatory and autoimmune neuropathies (e.g., Guillain-Barré syndrome and chronic inflammatory demyelinating polyneuropathy)
   - Infectious neuropathies (e.g., leprosy, Lyme disease)
   - Nutritional neuropathies (e.g., vitamin B12 or thiamine deficiency)
   - Idiopathic neuropathy (cause unknown)
   - Malignancy (e.g., paraprotein-associated neuropathies such as amyloidosis, multiple myeloma, POEMS syndrome (**P**olyneuropathy, **O**rganomegaly, **E**ndocrinopathy, **M**onoclonal gammopathy, **S**kin changes)

E. *Classification Based on **Nerve Cell Component**, e.g.,* **Axonal Neuropathy** *vs* **Demyelinating Neuropathy**. *Some diseases can affect both axon and myelin.*

### *Diagnosis of Peripheral Neuropathy*

**History:** Peripheral neuropathies often present in a "glove-and-stocking" distribution:

- The patient may report a "pins-and-needles" sensation (paresthesias) in the hands or feet if there is a sensory neuropathy.
- The report may include muscle weakness or cramping, particularly in the distal extremities,

- If there is an autonomic neuropathy, there may be abnormal sweating, bowel or bladder dysfunction, orthostatic dizziness, or sexual dysfunction.
- There may be a history of *systemic disease* (e.g., diabetes, renal failure, thyroid disorders, or autoimmune disease), exposure to *toxins* (e.g., alcohol abuse, chemotherapy, heavy metals), *nutritional deficiency* (e.g., vitamin B12, thiamine, folate), or a *family history* (e.g., Charcot-Marie-Tooth disease, familial amyloidosis). *Chronic infection, inflammation, malignancy*, or *trauma* may point to an underlying cause and treatment.

**Physical Exam:** Assess sensory deficits, motor strength, deep tendon reflexes, and autonomic function (blood pressure for orthostatic hypotension; heart rate).

**Lab Tests:** Blood tests for glucose levels, HbA1c, vitamins B1 and B12, thyroid function tests, serum protein electrophoresis (some monoclonal gammopathies can be associated with peripheral neuropathy), erythrocyte sedimentation rate (for inflammation), and antinuclear antibody titers (for autoimmune disorders that may be associated with peripheral neuropathy, e.g., lupus, Sjögren's syndrome, rheumatoid arthritis).

**Electrodiagnostic Studies:** Nerve conduction studies and electromyography (EMG) can determine the distribution, severity, and type of nerve fiber involvement. This helps differentiate between axonal degeneration and demyelination. In axonal degeneration, the main problem is loss of nerve axons, leading to decreased amplitude of nerve conduction without significantly affecting nerve conduction velocity. In demyelinating neuropathies, nerve conduction studies show slowed conduction velocities, while the amplitude of the nerve conduction may be preserved (early in the disease). Nerve conduction studies, EMG, ultrasound, and MRI are all techniques that can be used in confirming carpal tunnel syndrome.

**Cerebral spinal fluid (CSF) analysis** for signs of inflammation, infection, autoimmune disease, or malignancy. This can help if there is suspicion of a neuropathy that also involves the central nervous system, e.g., multiple sclerosis; Guillain-Barré syndrome; neurosyphilis; Lyme disease; sarcoidosis; lupus; Sjögren's syndrome; vasculitic neuropathies (increased CSF protein without significant increase in white blood cells); paraneoplastic syndromes (specific antibodies or inflammatory markers suggesting an immune response to cancer elsewhere in the body); mitochondrial diseases (elevated CSF lactate); leukodystrophies (progressive degeneration of brain white matter, which may have elevated CSF protein levels).

**Genetic testing** may be Indicated when a hereditary neuropathy is suspected, such as Charcot-Marie-Tooth disease.

**Nerve biopsy** is reserved for cases where the diagnosis remains unclear or there is a question of vasculitic or amyloid neuropathy.

### *Treatment of Peripheral Neuropathy*

Management of underlying conditions is key. This includes tight glycemic control in diabetic neuropathy, supplementation in nutritional deficiencies, and immunomodulatory therapies for autoimmune causes.

**Symptomatic Management:**

- **Pharmacotherapy** for neuropathic pain includes OTC pain medications (e.g., acetaminophen, NSAIDs, or opioids sometimes), anticonvulsants (e.g., *pregabalin, gabapentin*), antidepressants (e.g., *amitriptyline*), serotonin-norepinephrine reuptake inhibitors (e.g., *duloxetine*), and topical treatments (e.g., *capsaicin cream*). Treatment

of autonomic symptoms may include pharmacotherapy for orthostatic hypotension or gastrointestinal dysmotility. *Vutrisiran* reduces the production of the transthyretin protein responsible for amyloid buildup, which can cause a polyneuropathy.
- **Physical therapy and rehabilitation** can help maintain muscle strength and function, prevent contractures, and improve balance.
- **Surgical treatment** may be recommended to relieve nerve entrapment and compression (e.g., **carpal tunnel syndrome** or **ulnar nerve compression**) when conservative measures are not adequate, such as splinting, NSAIDs, corticosteroid injection, ergonomic changes, or physical therapy.

**Lifestyle modifications** include smoking cessation, foot care in diabetic patients, optimal diet, and avoidance of exacerbating factors.

**Emerging therapies** for peripheral neuropathy include newer drugs for neuropathic pain, immunomodulatory drugs to combat immune attack on peripheral nerves, gene therapy for hereditary neuropathies like Charcot-Marie-Tooth disease, stem cell therapy to assist in the regeneration of peripheral nerves, spinal cord stimulation or transcutaneous electrical nerve stimulation (TENS) for neuropathic pain, and monoclonal antibodies to target specific aspects of the inflammatory pathways.

## Carpal Tunnel Syndrome

In **carpal tunnel syndrome**, the patient may report numbness, tingling, and pain in the thumb, index, middle, and part of the ring finger, along with weakness in grip strength and muscle cramping, due to median nerve compromise in the carpal tunnel of the wrist (**Fig. 10-2**). The condition often arises from repetitive hand use, but risk factors also include other conditions that may cause swelling or inflammation in the wrist, such as rheumatoid arthritis, hypothyroidism, obesity, diabetes, or heredity. **Tinel's sign** (lightly tapping on the median nerve at the wrist to see if it causes tingling of the fingers) and **Phalen's maneuver** (holding the wrists flexed for about a minute to see if this induces symptoms) are diagnostic tests. In **ulnar neuropathy**, most commonly from compression of the ulnar nerve at the elbow, the patient reports numbness, tingling, or pain in the ulnar distribution to the little finger, inner half of the ring finger and part of the palm and back of the hand (**Fig. 10-2**).

Conservative treatment of carpal tunnel consists of wrist splinting (especially at night, when symptoms are commonly worse), physical therapy, and NSAIDs or corticosteroid injections. If this doesn't work, surgical intervention may be recommended (carpal tunnel release). Ulnar neuropathy is treated similarly, with bracing (of the elbow), physical therapy, NSAIDs or corticosteroid injections, and surgery if needed to relieve pressure on the ulnar nerve.

## Post-Herpetic Neuralgia

Post-herpetic neuralgia is persistent pain or sensitivity to touch or temperature along a dermatome as a residue of shingles (*herpes zoster*), an attack of chickenpox virus the second time around. While the blistery rash of shingles subsides over about 2-4 weeks, post-herpetic neuralgia may persist for weeks to years. The pain may be described as burning, sharp, aching, itchy or tingling. The affected area may show some residual rash, scarring, or change in skin color. Treatment may include anticonvulsants, e.g., *gabapentin* (*Neurontin*), *pregabalin* (*Lyrica*) for nerve pain; antidepressants; analgesics; or topical agents (e.g., *capsaicin* cream, *lidocaine* patches or cream) for pain.

## Phantom Pain

Phantom pain is the sensation of pain coming from a body part that is no longer present, generally following amputation. It is not simply stump pain but a feeling that the entire body part is still there, and painful. Although the body part is gone, its representation in the brain is still there.

Medications to treat phantom pain include antidepressants (e.g., *amitriptyline*), anticonvulsants (e.g., *gabapentin, pregabalin*), NSAIDs or opioids, and beta blockers and calcium channel blockers, which can reduce sympathetic nervous system activity and help relieve anxiety. Phantom pain can also be treated with nerve blocks, physical therapy exercises, massage, and cognitive-behavioral therapy.

## Complex Regional Pain Syndrome

Complex regional pain syndrome is a severe, chronic pain, sometimes feeling like burning or "pins-and-needles," usually in an arm or leg and disproportionate to any injury that may have occurred. The mechanism is unclear but seems to involve some sort of malfunction of signaling in the peripheral and central nervous systems. It may occur with confirmed nerve damage (*causalgia*) or without confirmed nerve damage (*reflex sympathetic dystrophy*). Symptoms may last months or years or fluctuate. Diagnosis depends largely on the exclusion or other conditions. Treatment may include pain medications; physical therapy; intravenous ketamine to help reduce pain, partly by blocking pain signals; spinal cord or peripheral nerve stimulation to mask pain signals; psychotherapy; and sometimes sympathetic nerve block. (Sympathetic nerve signals can contribute to pain by inducing changes in blood flow, inflammation, and pain sensitivity.) Some people report relief from alternative therapies, such as acupuncture, biofeedback, or transcutaneous electrical nerve stimulation (TENS) near the painful area.

## Syringomyelia

Syringomyelia is a condition where a cyst (**syrinx**) forms in the center of the spinal cord, usually in the upper cervical region. Although syringomyelia can cause loss of pain-temperature sensation in a "cape-like" distribution due to damage to the crossing pain-temperature fibers in the spinal cord (**Fig. 3-5F**), in some people it can cause pain, rather than loss of pain. The pain can be dull, aching, or throbbing but can also present as burning, stabbing, shooting, tingling, or numbness. Syringomyelia can also affect segmental muscle strength if the syrinx is large enough to affect peripheral motor fibers at that level.

Treatment of syringomyelia is mainly symptomatic, although surgery can sometimes help when there is a **Chiari malformation**, where cerebellar tissue extends into the spinal canal, causing pressure on the spinal cord. It may be possible to relieve this pressure surgically through decompression.

## Central Pain Syndrome

Central Pain Syndrome (CPS) is a chronic pain condition that arises within the central nervous system (CNS), e.g., from stroke, multiple sclerosis, spinal cord injury, or brain trauma. The pain is often described as constant, intensely painful, sometimes burning, stabbing, or shooting, and can be exacerbated by touch, movement, emotions, and temperature changes.

*Diagnosis of Central Pain Syndrome*

**History and Physical Exam:** Is there a history or any evidence on exam of damage to the CNS? If so, where is it located?

**Imaging:** MRI or CT scans may be able to see the abnormality.

**Neuropsychological Evaluation:** To help assess the degree to which the pain impacts the patient's life

*Treatment of Central Pain Syndrome*

**Medication:**

- **Anticonvulsants** (e.g., *gabapentin, pregabalin*) may help manage neuropathic pain.
- **Antidepressants** (e.g., *amitriptyline, duloxetine*) may help manage pain and accompanying depression.
- **Analgesics**: NSAIDs or limited use of opioids in some cases

**Physical Therapy:** May include massage, heat and cold therapy, or electrical nerve stimulation

**Cognitive Behavioral Therapy (CBT):** Helps with coping strategies to deal with chronic pain and stress management

**Neuromodulation Techniques:** Spinal cord stimulation (SCS) through an implanted device to interfere with pain transmission to the spinal cord and brain, or deep brain stimulation (DBS) through electrodes implanted in the brain may help some patients by modulating pain signals.

**Surgery:** In some cases, where the pain is localized, surgical procedures can target dorsal motor roots where pain fibers enter the spinal cord.

## Restless Legs Syndrome

Restless legs syndrome is characterized by abnormal sensations (creeping, crawling, itching, tingling, or pulling) in the legs and an uncomfortable urge to move them. It improves with activity and is worse at night. The condition is probably caused by dysfunction of the dopaminergic system and possibly iron deficiency in the brain (iron is needed in dopamine production). It can run in families.

*Diagnosis of Restless Legs Syndrome*

The diagnosis rests in part on the history, but blood tests and nerve conduction or imaging studies may be done to rule out other conditions that may mimic it in ways (e.g., peripheral neuropathy; leg cramps; peripheral artery or venous disease).

*Treatment of Restless Legs Syndrome*

**Lifestyle Modifications**: Establish a regular sleep schedule; exercise; relaxation techniques; avoid caffeine, alcohol, tobacco, and any drugs that might act as a trigger.

**Medications**:

- Dopamine agonists (e.g., *pramipexole* or *ropinirole*)
- Anticonvulsants (e.g., *gabapentin, pregabalin*) help stabilize nerve signaling.
- Iron supplements for people with low iron. Low blood levels of ferritin can help establish iron deficiency.
- Opioids may help some people who are refractive to other measures by relief of discomfort, sedative effect, or direct CNS action by dampening abnormal motor activity.

Some people report benefit from massage, hot or cold packs, or alternative treatments such as acupuncture or chiropractic.

# 21

# Seizures

Seizures are sudden, uncontrolled electrical disturbances in the brain that can manifest as changes in behavior, movements, feelings, and levels of consciousness. They occur in epilepsy but can also happen in other conditions such as fever, brain injury, infections, or metabolic imbalances (**Fig. 21-1**).

Seizures can be focal (partial) or generalized:

**Focal Aware Seizures (Simple Partial Seizures)**, typically unilateral, are those where the patient remains conscious during the seizure, which only involves a small part of one brain hemisphere. There may be twitching, changes in emotion, e.g., fear, depression, euphoria, anger, déjà vu, jamais vu (lack of familiarity with a place, person, or situation that should be familiar), visual disturbances (e.g., flashing lights), or altered autonomic function (e.g., changes in heart rate, sweating, pupillary dilation, hyperventilation, nausea, and increased blood pressure).

**Focal Impaired Awareness Seizures (complex partial seizures)** are focal seizures where consciousness is impaired during the seizure. There may be a preceding aura, which the patient may remember, and a postictal state of sleepiness and confusion.

**Generalized seizures**, which simultaneously involve both sides of the brain, include:

**Absence Seizures (petit mal)**: Involve brief sudden lapses in attention for seconds, generally in childhood.

**Atonic Seizures**: Sudden loss of muscle tone, typically bilateral, and collapse

**Tonic-Clonic Seizures (grand mal):** Bilateral stiffening of the body (the tonic part) followed by muscle jerks (the clonic part). They usually last about 1-3 minutes, with loss of consciousness, followed by a postictal state (confusion, fatigue, memory problems,

**FIGURE 21-1. CAUSES OF SEIZURES**

**Epilepsy**
Idiopathic Epilepsy
Symptomatic Epilepsy (associated with brain abnormalities, e.g., tumors, AV malformations, cerebral palsy)

**Acute Medical Conditions Associated with Seizures**
Febrile Seizures
Infections (e.g., meningitis, encephalitis, cerebral malaria)
Stroke, TIA
Brain Injury

**Developmental Disorders Associated with Seizures**
Autism Spectrum Disorder (often with problems with social communication and interaction; restricted or repetitive behaviors)
Tuberous Sclerosis (a genetic disorder with growth of benign tumors in multiple organs, including the brain)
Sturge-Weber (a mutation that causes angiomas of the meninges, as well as a facial port-wine stain. It can lead to seizures, stroke-like symptoms, intellectual disability, and headaches.)
Genetic Epilepsy Syndromes:

- Juvenile Myoclonic Epilepsy
- Childhood Absence Epilepsy
- Dravet Syndrome (a severe epilepsy in infancy, with frequent prolonged seizures often triggered by fever or heat, with developmental delays and other neurological issues)
- Lennox-Gastaut Syndrome (a severe childhood epilepsy with multiple types of seizures, cognitive dysfunction, and a distinctive EEG pattern)

Mitochondrial Disorders (e.g., MELAS – **M**itochondrial **E**ncephalomyopathy, **L**actic **A**cidosis, and **S**troke-like episodes)

**Metabolic and Electrolyte Imbalances Associated with Seizures**
Hypoglycemia
Hepatic Encephalopathy
Uremic Encephalopathy

**Toxic Causes of Seizures**
Alcohol Withdrawal
Drug Abuse or Withdrawal
Poisoning (e.g., lead, carbon monoxide, insecticides)

**Other Causes of Seizures**
Autoimmune Disorders (e.g., lupus, antiphospholipid syndrome, autoimmune encephalitis)
Medications (e.g., antidepressants, antipsychotics, stimulants, certain antibiotics; withdrawal from benzodiazepines, barbiturates)
Sleep-related Epilepsy (can happen at any stage of sleep)
Psychogenic Causes (resemble seizures but are psychogenic without EEG findings indicative of epilepsy)
Migraine with Aura

headache, speech difficulty, or motor weakness [**Todd's paralysis**]). Some seizures can be individually tonic, causing a person to fall; others can be individually clonic.

**Myoclonic seizures** are sudden, brief jerks of a muscle or group of muscles, typically bilateral, lasting about 1-2 seconds. There is no loss of consciousness or postictal state.

Focal seizures, typically unilateral, can evolve into generalized seizures, typically bilateral, which involve all areas of the brain.

In **temporal lobe epilepsy**, the patient may have a wide range of symptoms, including déjà vu (a sense of familiarity); jamais vu (a sense of unfamiliarity with something that should be very familiar); sudden feelings of fear, panic, or happiness; auditory or visual hallucinations; unusual smells or tastes; cognitive dysfunction; personality changes; inappropriate social behavior; or other seizure manifestations.

*Diagnosis of Seizures*

**History** should include the seizure manifestations, precipitating factors, frequency, duration, and any associated prodromal symptoms or postictal states. Precipitation factors can include missed antiepileptic medication, sleep deprivation, stress, fever, drug abuse or withdrawal, flashing lights, hormonal changes, hypoglycemia, heat, overexertion, medication interactions, and flickering screens. If there were witnesses to the event, inquire about what they noticed. A family history of seizures or epilepsy should also be documented, if available.

**Physical Exam:** Are there signs of tongue bite, incontinence, or injuries sustained during the fall? Does the patient show postictal confusion or drowsiness, as is common after a generalized tonic-clonic seizure? Once the patient is conscious, does the neurologic exam suggest any postictal neurological deficits, which might suggest a focal origin of the seizure?

**EEG:** Apart from confirming a seizure, the different forms of epilepsy show different patterns on EEG. Prolonged EEG monitoring may be needed to capture seizure events, as they are not always readily seen.

**Imaging:** MRI with epilepsy protocol (enhanced T1, T2, or FLAIR sequences) may identify structural brain abnormalities that may be causing seizures. CT scans may be used when MRI is contraindicated or unavailable. PET and SPECT scans can further assist in localizing seizure foci, especially in pre-surgical evaluation.

**Lab Tests:** E.g., blood glucose, electrolytes, calcium and magnesium, liver and renal function tests, blood ammonia, arterial blood gases, toxicology, lactate and pyruvate, thyroid function tests, and CBC can exclude metabolic causes of seizures, evaluate for infectious etiologies, and assess for potential toxic exposures. Genetic testing may be considered, depending on the seizure type and family history.

*Treatment of Seizures*

**Pharmacotherapy:** Antiepileptic drugs are chosen based on the type of seizures, patient age, comorbidities, and potential side effects. Monotherapy is preferred initially, with adjustments or additions based on efficacy and tolerability.

For **focal seizures**, *carbamazepine, phenytoin, levetiracetam, lamotrigine, oxcarbazepine, gabapentin, pregabalin, topiramate*, or *zonisamide* are treatment options.

For **generalized seizures**, *valproate, lamotrigine, levetiracetam, topiramate* or *zonisamide* are choices.

For **absence seizures**, *ethosuximide, valproate*, or *lamotrigine* may be beneficial.

For **myoclonic seizures**, *valproate* or *levetiracetam* are options.

For **temporal lobe epilepsy**: *Carbamazepine, lamotrigine, levetiracetam*, or *oxcarbazepine*

**Dravet Syndrome**: *Stiripentol, cannabidiol, fenfluramine, clobazam, valproate, topiramate, levetiracetam,* and ketogenic diet (stabilizes brain's electrical activity by shifting from glucose to ketone bodies for fuel)

**Lennox-Gastaut Syndrome**: *Valproate, lamotrigine, clobazam, rufinamide, topiramate, felbamate, cannabidiol;* ketogenic diet

For **mitochondrial disorders**: *Levetiracetam, lamotrigine, zonisamide*

For **pregnancy**: *Lamotrigine* and *levetiracetam* are preferred due to lower risk of teratogenic effects.

For **elderly patients**: *Gabapentin, lamotrigine,* and *levetiracetam* have a lower risk of side effects.

**Surgery:** When seizures are drug-resistant, surgical options include resective surgery, laser ablation, corpus callosotomy (prevents spread of seizures from one hemisphere to the other), or hemispherectomy, based on the seizure focus and functional brain mapping.

**Diet:** Includes the ketogenic diet, modified Atkins diet, or low glycemic index treatment for drug-resistant cases, especially in children. Switching from glucose to ketones for energy has been shown to stabilize neuronal activity and reduce seizure susceptibility.

**Neuromodulation:** For epilepsy that cannot be controlled by medication or surgery, several forms of neuromodulation may be effective in some individuals:

- **Vagus Nerve Stimulation**: A device is implanted that delivers electrical impulses to the vagus nerve in the neck. These impulses transmit to the brain, where they can help decrease the frequency and intensity of seizures.
- **Responsive Neurostimulation**: A neurostimulator device, implanted in the skull, monitors brain activity and delivers electrical stimulation directly to the seizure focus when it detects abnormal electrical patterns that precede a seizure.
- **Deep Brain Stimulation**: Surgical electrodes are implanted in the brain, e.g., the thalamus. A pacemaker-like device delivers electrical impulse to modulate the activity of brain regions involved in seizures.
- **Transcranial Magnetic Stimulation**: Magnetic fields stimulate neurons in specific areas of the brain. This may reduce seizure frequency in some individuals.
- **Trigeminal Nerve Stimulation**: Electrical stimulation of the trigeminal nerve through the skin and (like vagus nerve stimulation) may be used in some individuals with drug-resistant epilepsy not amenable to surgery.

**Emergency Management of a Seizure:** Treating an epilepsy attack in public has several guiding principles:

- **Stay calm** and reassure any bystanders. Check for a medical ID bracelet or necklace that may provide information about the individual's condition.
- **Ensure Safety**: Gently guide the person to the ground to prevent a fall. Put something soft behind the head (e.g., a jacket) to prevent head injury. Clear the area of any hard or sharp objects. Do not attempt to restrain the person's movements or put anything into the patient's mouth.
- **Time the seizure**: If it's longer than 5 minutes or there are multiple seizures without regaining consciousness between them call emergency services immediately.

- **Position the person**: If possible, gently turn the person onto the side, to prevent choking from fluid or vomit.
- **Stay with the person** until the seizure ends and he or she is fully conscious. Be reassuring and explain to the patient what has happened.
- **Call for emergency** if the seizure lasts longer than 5 minutes; another seizure starts after the first one ends; the person does not regain consciousness or has difficulty breathing after the seizure ends; the person is injured during the seizure; you know it is the person's first seizure; or the person has a health condition like diabetes, heart disease, or is pregnant. Do not try to prevent tongue biting by placing any object in the person's mouth; it may cause broken teeth, airway obstruction, or a bite risk to the rescuer.
- **After the seizure**, help the person sit in a safe place until fully recovered.
- **Be supportive and reassuring.**

In a hospital setting:
- Check glucose (hypoglycemia can cause seizures)
- For a first seizure workup:
  - CT scan of head (rule out structural cause)
  - Basic labs (glucose, sodium, calcium)
  - Toxicology screen
  - Neurology consult

For a known epileptic with a seizure:
- Check medication levels
- Look for triggers (missed doses, infection, sleep deprivation)
- Usually can discharge if back to baseline

Seizure Red Flags:
- Status epilepticus (>5 minutes)
- First seizure in adult
- Focal neurologic deficits after seizure
- Fever with seizure
- Head trauma history

When available, intravenous antiepileptic drugs may be administered to rapidly control a severe seizure. These include **benzodiazepines** (*lorazepam [Ativan], diazepam [Valium]*), **barbiturates** (*phenobarbital*); or **other drugs** - *Levetiracetam (Deppra), phenytoin (Dilantin),* or *valproate (Depacon).*

# 22

# Abnormal Movements

"Abnormal movements" encompasses a wide range of disorders, including Parkinson's disease, essential tremor, dystonia, chorea, tics, myoclonus, and ataxia. Many of them involve the basal ganglia or cerebellum in some way.

The Basics:
TREMOR:
- At rest = Parkinson's disease
- With movement = Essential tremor, cerebellar disease
- Action: Neurology referral (not emergency)

PARKINSON'S TRIAD:
- Tremor (at rest, "pill-rolling")
- Rigidity (stiff, "cogwheel")
- Bradykinesia (slow movement)
- Action: Neurology referral, trial of levodopa

CHOREA (Random Jerky Movements):
- Think: Huntington's disease, drug side effects
- Action: Neurology referral, medication review

DYSTONIA (Sustained Abnormal Postures):
- Think: Drug side effects, genetic
- Action: Stop offending drug, neurology referral

Movement Disorder Red Flags:
- Acute onset (drug reaction)
- With fever (neuroleptic malignant syndrome - a form of severe drug-induced parkinsonism / hypokinetic–rigid syndrome.)
- Difficulty swallowing / breathing
- Rapidly progressive

Simple Rule: Most movement disorders are not emergencies unless acute onset

Movement disorders can be classified into **hyperkinetic** (excess movements) and **hypokinetic** (reduced movement) **(Fig. 22-1).** Visual examples of each may be found on YouTube.

**FIGURE 22-1. MOVEMENT DISORDERS**

***Hyperkinetic Movement Disorders***

***Tremor*:** Rhythmic, oscillating movements of one or more parts of the body, most commonly in the hands but can affect other body parts. Tremor can occur at rest (**resting tremor**—basal ganglia origin) or during movement (**action tremor**—cerebellar origin). *Titubation* is an involuntary oscillation or trembling of the head, trunk or limbs.

**Causes of Tremor**

- Essential tremor: The most common movement disorder, usually in the hands, worsening when performing tasks (includes "yes-yes" or "no-no" head tremors while keeping the head up) (an action tremor—may relate to abnormal thalamic activity; may be familial)
- Parkinson's disease (resting tremor, involving degeneration of the midbrain substantia nigra, a part of the basal ganglia)
- Multiple sclerosis (action)
- Cerebellar disorders (action)
- Dystonic tremor (occurs in individuals with dystonia) (action)
- Hypothyroidism (action)
- Wilson's disease (a genetic disorder with copper accumulation in liver, brain, eyes, and other organs) (action or resting)
- Drug-induced (action or resting)
- Alcohol withdrawal (action)
- Psychogenic stress-related (action or resting)
- Orthostatic tremor (rapid tremors in the legs and sometimes the trunk when standing up) (action)
- Peripheral neuropathy (action)
- Hepatic encephalopathy (action—*asterixis* is a brief flapping tremor when the arms are outstretched and wrists bent upward)
- Stroke (action or resting)

***Athetosis:*** Slow, continuous, writhing movements that are often fluid and sinuous. Athetosis primarily affects the hands and feet but can involve other body parts. Movements are involuntary and can interfere with fine motor skills. (basal ganglia origin)

**Causes of Athetosis**

- Cerebral palsy
- Huntington's disease
- Wilson's disease
- Rett syndrome (a genetic condition with hand-wringing along with developmental disability)
- Kernicterus (a bilirubin-induced encephalopathy in infants)

***Chorea*:** Sudden, rapid, brief, non-repetitive, irregular involuntary movements that seem to move from one muscle to the next, particularly in the limbs or facial muscles. Can affect the face, mouth, trunk, and limbs. (basal ganglia origin)

**Causes of Chorea**

- Huntington's disease
- Sydenham's chorea (an autoimmune reaction triggered by untreated streptococcal infections, particularly rheumatic fever)
- Wilson's disease
- Benign hereditary chorea
- Neuroacanthocytosis syndromes—rare degenerative conditions with misshapen, spiky red blood cells (acanthocytes) and neurological abnormalities
- Drug-induced
- Hemichorea-hemiballism
- Lupus
- Pregnancy (*chorea gravidarum*—may be associated with underlying rheumatic fever or lupus)
- Certain metabolic disorders (hyperglycemia, hyperthyroidism, electrolyte imbalances) by affecting brain function
- Infections (HIV, bacterial endocarditis) due to inflammation affecting the basal ganglia

***Tardive dyskinesia*:** Choreoathetosis as a side effect of long-term use or abrupt discontinuation of certain dopamine blocking agents, including the older antipsychotic medications like *haloperidol* and *chlorpromazine*

***Dystonia*:** Sustained or intermittent muscle contractions causing abnormal, often repetitive, twisting movements, or postures that can affect any part of the body. Movements are typically patterned and can be worsened by voluntary actions. Some forms are inherited. (basal ganglia origin)

**Causes of Dystonia**

- Drug side effect
- Idiopathic torsion dystonia
- DYT1 dystonia (a hereditary condition usually beginning in childhood or adolescence)
- Spasmodic torticollis
- Blepharospasm (Involuntary, forceful contractions of the eyelids)
- Oromandibular dystonia
- Writer's cramp
- Parkinson's disease (along with bradykinesia, tremor, and rigidity)
- Huntington's disease
- Wilson's disease
- Traumatic brain injury
- Stroke
- Cerebral palsy
- Certain metabolic disorders, infections, and autoimmune disorders

- Tetanus (muscle spasms and rigidity from tetanus toxin)
- Rabies (may resemble dystonia as it includes muscle spasms and rigidity)
- Stiff Person Syndrome: A rare disorder of fluctuating muscle rigidity and painful spasms in the trunk and limbs

***Myoclonus*:** Sudden, brief, involuntary non-rhythmic shock-like twitching or jerking of a muscle or group of muscles, which can vary in intensity and frequency. It can occur spontaneously or in response to an external stimulus. (cerebral cortex, brain stem, or spinal cord origin)

**Causes of Myoclonus**
- Alzheimer's disease
- Creutzfeldt-Jakob disease
- Parkinson's disease
- Lewy body dementia
- Juvenile myoclonic epilepsy
- Progressive myoclonic epilepsies (seizures with a progressive decline in movement and cognition)
- Hepatic encephalopathy
- Uremia
- Electrolyte imbalances (calcium, magnesium, sodium) (due to altered neuronal excitability):
  - Hypocalcemia (tetany, with muscle cramps, spasms, or tremors)
  - Hypercalcemia (muscle weakness)
  - Hypomagnesemia (tremors, muscle spasms, cramps, and tetany)
  - Hypermagnesemia (muscle weakness)
  - Hyponatremia (brain swelling, with headaches, seizures, and sometimes coma)
  - Hypernatremia (muscle twitching and spasms)
- Viral encephalitis
- Subacute sclerosing panencephalitis (a chronic progressive encephalitis in children or young adults from persistent mutant measles virus. Can cause movement disorders, cognitive decline, seizures, motor and autonomic dysfunction, and coma)
- Certain antidepressants, antipsychotics and antibiotics
- Certain toxins (carbon monoxide, heavy metals)
- Hypoxia
- Stroke or brain injury
- Multiple system atrophy (a progressive neurodegenerative disorder of the brain and spinal cord that affects autonomic function, movement, and coordination)
- Hypnic myoclonus (sudden jerks when transitioning from wakefulness to sleep, generally considered benign)

***Tics*:** Sudden, rapid, repetitive, stereotyped, nonrhythmic motor movements or (sometimes obscene) vocalizations. They can be simple or complex and are often preceded by an urge or sensation. Tics can be temporarily voluntarily suppressed. These can be simple, involving a limited number of muscles, or complex, involving coordinated movements or phrases. (basal ganglia origin)

**Causes of Tics**
- Tourette's syndrome (tics may be motor or vocal or involve a complex mixture of the two)
- Persistent chronic motor or vocal tic disorders
- Provisional tic disorder (motor or vocal tics in children lasting less than one year from the time first noted)
- Autism spectrum disorder

- Medications for Attention Deficit Hyperactivity Disorder (e.g., *Ritalin, Adderall, Vyvanse*)
- Other drugs (e.g., antipsychotics, antiepileptics, cocaine, excess caffeine, Selective Serotonin Reuptake Inhibitors)
- Post-streptococcal
- Psychogenic

***Hemiballismus*:** Sudden, wild, flinging movements of the limbs on one side of the body. It is caused by damage to the contralateral subthalamic nucleus of the basal ganglia. The movements are violent and can be exhausting for the patient.

**Causes of Hemiballismus**

- Stroke
- Traumatic brain injury
- Autoimmune disorders causing blood vessel inflammation
- Nonketotic hyperglycemia
- Brain tumors, cysts, or AV malformations near the subthalamic nucleus
- Infectious disorders of the brain
- Autoimmune disorders (lupus, cerebral vasculitis)
- Toxins (carbon monoxide or manganese poisoning)
- Parkinson's disease (as a medication side effect)

***Hypokinetic Movement Disorders***

**Parkinson's Disease**: Slow movement, rigidity, or resting tremor, in any combination.

**Parkinsonism**: Same symptoms as Parkinson's disease but caused by drug side effects, brain damage, or other neurodegenerative diseases

**Progressive Supranuclear Palsy**: Problems walking, balance, eye movements (difficulty initiating eye movements, vertical gaze palsy, blepharospasm, nystagmus), early cognitive impairment, and, in later stages, rigid features like Parkinson's disease. (Origin in substantia nigra, subthalamic nucleus, other areas of the basal ganglia, brain stem nuclei, and prefrontal cortex)

**Multiple System Atrophy**: Autonomic dysfunction (orthostatic hypotension, urinary incontinence or difficulty initiating urination, sexual dysfunction, GI problems, excess or reduced sweating), sleep apnea, parkinsonism, and ataxia (poorly coordinated movement). (Origin in basal ganglia, cerebellum, brain stem, and parts of the autonomic nervous system)

**Corticobasal Degeneration**: Problems with movement (asymmetric rigidity and bradykinesia), apraxia, speech (aphasia), memory, and swallowing (dysphagia), and may include signs of dystonia, myoclonus, and tremor. (Origin in cerebral cortex and basal ganglia)

*Diagnosis of Movement Disorders*

**History**: Important aspects include the onset, duration, and progression of symptoms; triggers and alleviating factors; medication history; and any family history of neurological disorders.

**Distinguishing Features:**

**Speed:** *Athetosis* is slower than chorea and tremor.

**Rhythm:** *Tremor* is rhythmic, unlike the irregular movements of *athetosis* and *chorea.*

**Control:** *Dystonia* and *athetosis* both involve sustained movements, but dystonia is more likely to result in abnormal postures.

**Suddenness:** *Myoclonus* and *hemiballismus* are characterized by sudden movements, unlike the continuous flow of *athetosis*.

**Volition:** *Tics* can be temporarily suppressed, which is not typical for involuntary movements of *athetosis*.

**Imaging**: MRI or CT scans are important for identifying structural abnormalities that may contribute to abnormal movements, such as stroke, tumor, or atrophy. Functional imaging, like PET or SPECT, can be helpful by detecting changes in brain metabolism or neurotransmitter activity.

**Lab Tests**: Routine blood tests (e.g., CBC; electrolyte and metabolic panels; liver, kidney, and thyroid function tests) can identify infectious or metabolic problems that might contribute to movement disorders. Specific tests may include ceruloplasmin levels for Wilson's disease, and genetic testing for conditions like Huntington's disease and familial Parkinson's disease.

**Electrophysiological Studies**: EMG, nerve conduction studies, evoked potentials, and EEG can help differentiate muscle, peripheral nerve, or central origins of movement disorders.

**Response to Therapy**: In some cases, response to specific medications can be diagnostic, such as the dramatic improvement in motor symptoms with levodopa in Parkinson's disease.

### *Treatment of Parkinson's Disease*

Parkinson's disease classically is manifest as bilateral resting tremor, slowness and stiffness, with cogwheel rigidity (feels like a ratchety cogwheel on flexing or extending the wrist), decreased arm swing when walking, freezing (interruption in the ability to move forward), festinating gait (short, rapid shuffling steps), and micrographia (small handwriting). The face commonly has a masked, expressionless appearance, even though this may not reflect the patient's mood. Any of these can occur individually or unilaterally in early stages and need to be considered in treatment. Parkinson's disease affects about 1% of the population over the age of 60.

**Medications:**

**Levodopa/Carbidopa:** The primary treatment for Parkinson's disease symptoms, including tremor. Carbidopa increases the availability of levodopa to the brain by preventing the peripheral conversion of levodopa to dopamine, which does not cross the blood-brain barrier. The treatment is symptomatic and is given when the disease begins to interfere with daily activities.

**Dopamine agonists** (*pramipexole, ropinirole,* and *rotigotine*) directly stimulate dopamine receptors in the brain, mimicking dopamine.

**MAO-B inhibitors** (e.g., *selegiline, rasagiline, safinamide*) act by blocking the enzyme monoamine oxidase-B, which plays a role in breaking down neurotransmitters like dopamine.

**Catechol-O-methyltransferase (COMT) inhibitors** (e.g., *entacapone, tolcapone*) also act by inhibiting the breakdown of dopamine.

**Anticholinergic medications** (e.g., *trihexyphenidyl, benztropine [Cogentin]*) can be effective for tremor control but can have significant side effects (confusion, memory impairment, urinary retention, constipation, dry mouth, blurred vision), especially in older patients.

*Amantadine*, originally an anti-viral drug serendipitously found to help Parkinsonism, can provide short-term relief of mild, early-stage Parkinsonism and **dyskinesia** (erratic, writhing movements) that may occur with long-term levodopa use. Amantadine may act in part by antagonizing brain glutamate, an excitatory neurotransmitter.

The various drugs for Parkinson's disease can be used individually or in combination. Medication dose and timing are critical as symptoms over time may need a different treatment schedule due to "off" periods or side effects of drugs, e.g., dyskinetic (erratic, writhing) movements with levodopa.

**Deep brain stimulation (DBS)** may be recommended for patients with refractory symptoms. DBS involves surgical implantation of a neurostimulator into the brain when other treatments are not effective.

**Surgeries** (pallidotomy, thalamotomy) were more common before the widespread use of DBS.

**Rehabilitation**: Exercise, speech therapy if needed, and psychiatric treatment for depression, anxiety, or psychosis

*Treatment of Cerebellar Tremor*

**Medications:** *Isoniazid, beta-blockers,* and *anticonvulsants* might be tried, but medication effectiveness can be limited for cerebellar tremor.

**Surgical Treatments: Deep Brain Stimulation (DBS)** may be considered for severe cases.

## Treatment of Dystonic Tremor

**Medications:**

- Anticholinergics, beta-blockers, and anticonvulsants may provide some relief.
- **Botulinum Toxin Injections:** Can reduce tremors by temporarily paralyzing the overactive muscles causing the tremor

*Treatment of Orthostatic Tremor*

**Medications:** Benzodiazepines (*clonazepam*) and anticonvulsants (*gabapentin, pregabalin*) are commonly used.

**General Treatment Approaches:**

- **Physical Therapy:** Can help strengthen muscles and improve coordination and control, potentially reducing the impact of tremor on daily activities
- **Psychological Support:** Counseling or therapy can help manage the emotional and psychological impact of living with tremor.

## Treatment of Essential Tremor

**Medications**

- **Beta-Blockers:** *Propranolol* is commonly used to reduce tremor amplitude, especially in the hands. *Propranolol* blocks beta-adrenergic receptors, thereby decreasing the physiological response to adrenaline and noradrenaline.
- **Anticonvulsants:** *Primidone, gabapentin,* and *topiramate* may also be effective in reducing tremors.

- **Benzodiazepines:** Drugs like *clonazepam* can help reduce tremor in some patients but are generally used sparingly due to their potential for dependency and side effects.

**Lifestyle Modifications and Assistive Devices:** Adaptive devices (e.g., weighted utensils, braces, jar openers, writing aids, buttonhooks) and avoiding caffeine and other stimulants can help manage tremor effects on daily activities.

**Alcohol:** Small amounts of alcohol may temporarily reduce tremor in some individuals with essential tremor, though this is not recommended as a long-term treatment strategy due to the risks of alcohol misuse.

**Surgical Treatments:**

- **Deep Brain Stimulation (DBS):** Involves implanting electrodes in the thalamus, connected to a pulse generator placed in the chest to modulate the brain areas responsible for tremor
- **Focused Ultrasound Thalamotomy:** A non-invasive procedure that uses focused ultrasound waves to create lesions in the thalamus, reducing tremor

## Treatment of Athetosis

**Medications**

- **Anticholinergic Drugs:** Medications such as *trihexyphenidyl (Artane)* and *benztropine (Cogentin)* can help reduce involuntary movements by blocking the action of acetylcholine, a neurotransmitter that can be overactive in individuals with athetosis.
- **Dopaminergic Agents:** In some cases, medications that adjust dopamine levels in the brain, such as *levodopa* or dopamine *agonists*, might be used if there's an underlying dopamine imbalance contributing to the symptoms.
- **Muscle Relaxants:** Drugs like *baclofen (Lioresal)* and *tizanidine (Zanaflex)* may be prescribed to decrease muscle spasticity, which can co-occur with athetosis.
- **Benzodiazepines:** Medications like *clonazepam (Klonopin)* are sometimes used for their sedative and muscle relaxant properties to alleviate discomfort and reduce the severity of movements.

**Physical Therapy:** Aims to maintain or improve muscle strength and flexibility, which can help manage the involuntary movements and improve functional abilities

**Occupational Therapy:** Focuses on enhancing daily living skills, including the use of adaptive equipment or techniques to manage tasks at home, school, or work

**Surgical Interventions:**

- **Intrathecal Baclofen Pump:** A device that delivers *baclofen* directly to the spinal fluid, providing continuous muscle relaxation, which can be beneficial for those with severe spasticity as well as athetosis

**Deep Brain Stimulation (DBS):** In select cases, especially where athetosis is part of a broader movement disorder like Parkinson's disease or dystonia, DBS can be considered.

This involves surgically implanting electrodes in specific brain regions to modulate abnormal electrical signals.

**Selective Dorsal Rhizotomy (SDR):** While not specifically targeting athetosis, SDR can reduce spasticity in children with cerebral palsy and might indirectly improve overall movement control.

**Other Treatments:**

- **Speech Therapy:** For individuals whose athetosis affects the speech muscles, working with a speech-language pathologist can help improve communication abilities.
- **Adaptive Devices:** Tools and devices designed to assist with writing, eating, and other daily activities can improve independence and quality of life.

*Treatment of Chorea*

Treatment for chorea is primarily aimed at reducing the severity of the involuntary movements and improving the patient's quality of life. The approach varies depending on the underlying cause of the chorea:

**Medications**

- **Antipsychotics:** Antipsychotic medications, such as *haloperidol (Haldol)* and *risperidone (Risperdal)*, can be effective in reducing choreic movements by blocking dopamine receptors, which are often implicated in the pathophysiology of chorea.
- **Dopamine Depleters:** *Tetrabenazine (Xenazine)* and *deutetrabenazine (Austedo)* reduce dopamine levels in the brain and are specifically approved for the treatment of Huntington's disease-related chorea. They work by depleting presynaptic stores of dopamine and other monoamines from nerve terminals.
- **Benzodiazepines:** Drugs like *clonazepam (Klonopin)* can be used to treat chorea by enhancing the action of GABA, an inhibitory neurotransmitter, thereby reducing excessive neuronal firing.
- **Anticonvulsants:** Some antiepileptic drugs, such as *valproic acid (Depakote)* and *levetiracetam (Keppra)*, have been used off-label to manage chorea, possibly through stabilization of neuronal membranes and modulation of neurotransmitter release.

**Surgical and Other Interventions:**

**Deep Brain Stimulation (DBS):** In certain cases, especially for medically refractory chorea, DBS of the globus pallidus may be considered. DBS involves surgically implanting electrodes in specific brain areas to modulate abnormal electrical signals.

**Immunomodulatory Treatments:** For chorea resulting from autoimmune or post-infectious conditions (e.g., **Sydenham's chorea**), corticosteroids, intravenous immunoglobulins (IVIG), or plasmapheresis might be used to reduce inflammation and autoimmune activity.

**Physical Therapy:** Can help improve coordination and balance, reducing the risk of falls and helping patients manage daily activities more effectively

**Occupational Therapy:** Focuses on adapting the living and work environments to accommodate the patient's needs, thereby improving their ability to perform daily tasks

**Speech Therapy:** For those with chorea affecting speech and swallowing muscles, working with a speech therapist can help improve communication and reduce the risk of aspiration.

**Genetic Counseling:** In conditions like Huntington's disease, where chorea is a genetic disorder, genetic counseling is an important part of the management for the patient and his or her family.

**Treat Underlying Conditions** (e.g., infectious, autoimmune, vascular, drug-induced, or metabolic disorders)

Treatment of Tardive Dyskinesia

**Medication Adjustment**: Reduce the dose of the offending antipsychotic medication or switch to a different one (e.g., *clozapine* or *quetiapine*).

Use a **VMAT2 (Vesicular Monoamine Transporter 2) inhibitor**, such as *valbenazine* or *deutetrabenazine*, which decreases the action of dopamine on the hypersensitive dopamine receptors in tardive dyskinesia.

**Botulinum toxin** injections to target specific muscles involved in involuntary movements

**Supportive Therapy:** Physical, occupational, or speech therapy; psychosocial counseling or support groups

## Treatment of Dystonia

**Medications**

- **Botulinum Toxin Injections:** One of the most effective treatments for focal dystonias, such as cervical dystonia (neck), blepharospasm (eyelids), and writer's cramp (hand). Botulinum toxin (Botox) injections work by temporarily paralyzing the overactive muscles causing dystonia, thereby reducing symptoms. The effect usually lasts for about three months, after which the injections need to be repeated.
- **Oral Medications: Anticholinergics** (such as *trihexyphenidyl*) can help reduce muscle spasms by blocking acetylcholine, a neurotransmitter involved in muscle movement. *Baclofen* (a muscle relaxant) can reduce spasticity and muscle contractions. **Dopaminergic agents** (such as *levodopa*) for dopamine deficient dystonias, or dopamine-depleting medications (such as *tetrabenazine*) for dopamine excess dystonias, might be effective, depending on the kind of dopaminergic dysfunction. *Tetrabenazine*, which reduces the storage of monamine neurotransmitters like dopamine, is mainly used for treating hyperkinetic movement disorders (like Huntington's disease and chorea), while levodopa is primarily used for treating hypokinetic movement disorders (like Parkinson's disease). Dystonia, a hyperkinetic movement disorder, is sometime dopamine-responsive (e.g., in the rare childhood genetic disorder *dopa-responsive dystonia*).

**Physical Therapy:** Helps to maintain or improve muscle strength and flexibility, manage pain, and possibly reduce the severity of dystonia through stretching and strengthening exercises, as well as relaxation techniques

**Occupational Therapy:** Focuses on improving the ability to perform daily activities through adaptive strategies and equipment

**Surgical Treatments:**

- **Deep Brain Stimulation (DBS):** For patients with severe dystonia that is not adequately controlled by medications, DBS can be an option. It involves surgically implanting electrodes in specific areas of the brain connected to a pulse generator

placed in the chest. The generator sends electrical impulses to the brain to help control muscle contractions.
- **Selective Dorsal Rhizotomy:** In some cases, particularly for children with spastic dystonia primarily affecting the legs, this procedure can reduce muscle stiffness and improve mobility by cutting nerve fibers that contribute to muscle overactivity.

**Other Treatments**

- **Speech Therapy:** For those with dystonia affecting the jaw, tongue, or voice muscles, speech therapy can help improve communication abilities.
- **Stress Management and Relaxation Techniques:** Stress can often worsen dystonia symptoms, so techniques such as mindfulness, meditation, yoga, and biofeedback may help manage stress and reduce the severity of symptoms.

**Experimental Treatments:** Ongoing research into the causes and mechanisms of dystonia may lead to new treatments. Clinical trials investigating gene therapy, new medications, and other interventions offer hope for more effective treatments in the future.

## Treatment of Myoclonus

**Medications**

- **Anticonvulsants:** Drugs such as *levetiracetam (Keppra), valproic acid (Depakene, Depakote), clonazepam (Klonopin),* and *zonisamide (Zonegran)* are often effective in reducing myoclonic jerks. These medications stabilize electrical activity in the brain and can be helpful for various forms of myoclonus, especially those associated with epilepsy.
- **Barbiturates:** *Phenobarbital*, a barbiturate, can be used in certain cases, especially when myoclonus is part of a broader epileptic syndrome.
- **Benzodiazepines:** *Clonazepam (Klonopin)* is used for its effectiveness in treating several types of myoclonus. Benzodiazepines enhance the effect of the inhibitory neurotransmitter GABA and can help suppress myoclonic jerks.
- ***Piracetam*:** An adjunct therapy for myoclonus, especially cortical myoclonus. While its exact mechanism is not fully understood, *piracetam* is believed to reduce abnormal neuronal firing patterns.

**Non-Pharmacological Treatments:**

- **Lifestyle Adjustments:** Reducing caffeine and avoiding stimulants can help manage myoclonus. Adequate sleep and stress management may also reduce symptoms.
- **Physical Therapy:** Can help improve muscle control, coordination, and strength, potentially reducing the impact of myoclonus on daily activities
- **Surgical and Other Interventions:** In select cases, especially for severe, drug-resistant myoclonus, **Deep Brain Stimulation (DBS)** might be considered. This involves surgically implanting electrodes in specific brain regions that contribute to myoclonus to continuously deliver modulating electrical impulses to the targeted regions. **Responsive Neurostimulation (RNS)** involves a device that's implanted in the brain to monitor electrical activity and deliver electrical stimulation when abnormal patterns are detected.

**Treating Underlying Causes:** When myoclonus is secondary to another condition, treating the underlying cause is vital. This may involve:

- **Correcting Metabolic Imbalances:** For myoclonus due to metabolic or electrolyte imbalances, treatment focuses on correcting these abnormalities.
- **Immunotherapy:** For myoclonus caused by autoimmune conditions, treatments such as corticosteroids, intravenous immunoglobulins (IVIG), or plasmapheresis may be used.
- **Antibiotics or Antivirals:** If an infection is the underlying cause of myoclonus, appropriate antimicrobial therapy may alleviate the symptoms.

## Treatment of Tics

Treatment for tics depends on the severity of the tics and their impact on daily life. For many people with mild tics, treatment might not be necessary. However, when tics are severe, cause distress, or interfere with social, school, or work functioning, a combination of therapies may be recommended.

**Behavioral Therapies for Tics:**

**Comprehensive Behavioral Intervention for Tics (CBIT)** is a non-drug approach. It combines habit reversal training, education, and functional interventions to help manage tics. **Habit Reversal Training** by a behavioral therapist or psychologist teaches individuals to recognize the urge to tic and then perform a competing response that is incompatible with the tic. **Exposure and Response Prevention** involves gradually increasing exposure to the urge to tic without allowing the tic to occur, aiming to reduce the tic's frequency.

**Medications for Tics:** While there is no medication specifically designed to eliminate tics, several types may be used to help control them, especially when they're severe:

- **Antipsychotic Medications:** Anti-psychotics such as *risperidone (Risperdal)*, *aripiprazole (Abilify)*, and *haloperidol (Haldol)* can be effective in reducing tics but can have side effects, such as weight gain, sedation, and movement disorders, including tardive dyskinesia.
- **Alpha-2 Adrenergic Agonists:** Medications like *guanfacine (Intuniv)* and *clonidine (Catapres)* decrease the activity of norepinephrine and the sympathetic nervous system. They are often used as first-line treatments for tics due to their milder side effects compared to antipsychotics.
- **Botulinum Toxin Injections:** For adults with motor tics that involve specific muscle groups, botulinum toxin injections can help reduce the severity of tics by temporarily weakening the involved muscles.

**Supportive Therapies:**

- **Psychoeducation:** Educating the patient, family, teachers, and peers about tics can be an important part of treatment, reducing stigma and providing support.
- **Psychological Support:** Counseling or therapy can help individuals cope with the social and emotional challenges associated with having tics, such as anxiety or low self-esteem.

**Lifestyle and Home Remedies:**

- **Stress Management:** Since stress can exacerbate tics, techniques for stress reduction, such as mindfulness, meditation, and regular exercise, may help reduce tic frequency and severity.
- **Avoidance of Stimulants:** Stimulant substances, including caffeine, may worsen tics in some individuals and should be used cautiously.

*Treatment of Hemiballismus*

The treatment for hemiballismus focuses on reducing the severity of the movements and managing the underlying cause.

**Medications:**

- **Antipsychotics:** Dopamine receptor-blocking agents, such as *haloperidol* or other typical antipsychotics, can be effective in reducing hemiballistic movements by inhibiting dopamine pathways, which are believed to be overactive in hemiballismus.
- **Dopamine Depletors:** *Tetrabenazine*, a VMAT2 (Vesicular Monoamine Transporter 2) inhibitor, which depletes dopamine stores, reduces the activity in the subthalamic nucleus and can be used to control hemiballistic movements.
- **Anticonvulsants:** Medications like *valproic acid* and *carbamazepine*, which are traditionally used to treat epilepsy, have been used off-label to manage hemiballismus with varying degrees of success.
- **Benzodiazepines:** Drugs such as *clonazepam* may be used for their muscle-relaxant and sedative properties to help control the involuntary movements.
- **Botulinum toxin** injections into affected muscles can help reduce hemiballismus.

**Treating underlying causes,** e.g., stroke, infections, autoimmune disease, tumors, metabolic disorders, toxins, drug side effects (certain antipsychotics and dopamine-depleting medications)

**Deep Brain Stimulation (DBS)** of the globus pallidus or thalamus, or thalamotomy, may be considered as a treatment option in severe cases of hemiballismus that do not respond to medical therapy.

**Physical Therapy:** Can help improve muscle strength and coordination, potentially reducing the risk of injury caused by involuntary movements

**Occupational Therapy:** Aims to assist individuals in adapting their daily activities to manage the challenges posed by hemiballismus

**Safety Measures:** Implementing home safety measures to prevent injuries due to falls or the forceful movements associated with hemiballismus

*Treatment of Progressive Supranuclear Palsy*

**Parkinson's disease medication**, e.g., levodopa may temporarily improve stiffness and balance.

**Physical Therapy** for mobility

**Occupational Therapy**

**Speech and Language Therapy** for speech and swallowing difficulty

**Botulinum Toxin** injections for eyelid spasms

**Nutritional Support**

**Support Groups and Counseling**

*Treatment of Multiple System Atrophy*

**Parkinson's Disease Medications**

**Addressing autonomic dysfunction** with *fludrocortisone* (a corticosteroid that retains sodium) or *midodrine* (a vasoconstrictor) for orthostatic hypotension and *desmopressin* (promotes water reabsorption) for nocturnal polyuria

*Treatment of Corticobasal Degeneration*

**Parkinson's Disease Medications**

**Pain management** of dystonia and rigidity with analgesics, muscle relaxants, or botulinum toxin injections

**Speech therapy** for speech and swallowing problems

**Occupational Therapy**

**Support Groups**

## Stiff Person Syndrome (SPS)

Stiff Person Syndrome is somewhat difficult to classify. It is not primarily a disorder of weakness or movement, but one with progressive rigidity and painful spasms affecting the trunk and limbs, with impaired mobility and posture. It is believed due to autoimmune antibodies against *glutamic acid decarboxylase (GAD)* enzyme, which is needed to produce gamma-aminobutyric acid (GABA, the main inhibitory neurotransmitter in the brain), causing increased muscle tone and muscle spasms.

*Diagnosis of Stiff Person Syndrome (SPS)*

**Blood tests** can detect anti-GAD (glutamic acid decarboxylase) antibodies.

**EMG** can identify a pattern of rigidity and spasm characteristic of SPS.

**MRI** of the brain and spinal cord is used to rule out other conditions.

**Spinal tap** can show elevated GAD antibodies but are not specific for SPS. (They can also be found in type 1 diabetes, autoimmune encephalitis, some cerebellar ataxias, paraneoplastic, and other autoimmune neurological disorders, which may be related or coinciding.) The cerebrospinal fluid (CSF) can also show oligoclonal bands (immunoglobulins) indicating an immune response, but this again is not specific (can also be found in multiple sclerosis). CSF helps rule out infectious or inflammatory conditions, since the white cell count and protein levels are normal in SPS.

*Treatment of Stiff Person Syndrome*

The treatment focuses on managing muscle rigidity, spasticity, and pain to improve patient comfort, mobility, and function:

**NSAIDs** for milder pain, **opioids** for severe pain not adequately controlled by other means

**Muscle Relaxants**: Benzodiazepines can reduce muscle stiffness and spasm. *Baclofen* helps relax muscle by enhancing GABAergic action in the central nervous system.

**Anti-seizure Medications**: E.g., *gabapentin* or *pregabalin* to reduce spasm and pain

**Immunotherapy**: Intravenous immunoglobulins, plasmapheresis, or corticosteroids

**Physical Therapy**

## Tetanus

Tetanus presents with stiffness and spasms, particularly of the jaw (**lockjaw**) and neck muscles; difficulty swallowing; and **opisthotonos** (back muscle arching), often associated with wounds contaminated with *Clostridium tetani* bacteria. In severe cases there may be seizures, and spasms may be severe enough to cause bone fractures. There are no good diagnostic tests, and diagnosis depends largely on ruling out other diseases, a history of recent wounds, and inadequate vaccination. The treatment includes wound cleaning and tetanus immunoglobulin to neutralize any toxin that is not yet bound to neural tissue. Antibiotics, e.g. *metronidazole*, sometime *penicillin*, can be used to kill tetanus bacteria. Muscle relaxants and pain medication can help manage muscle spasms and pain. DTaP (Diphtheria, Tetanus, and Pertussis) vaccination may help if used during the acute phase.

# 23

# Balance and Coordination Problems

Problems with balance and coordination (**ataxia**) can arise in the central or peripheral nervous system (**Fig. 23-1**) and may be due to problems of muscle strength, proprioception, light touch, vestibular sense, vision, or cerebral or cerebellar dysfunction. They may also arise from drug effects, including alcohol. Some may have a genetic origin. Dizziness and vertigo are among the causes of ataxia and are discussed in **Chapter 19**.

Basic Causes of Balance Problems:

CAUSE 1: Inner Ear (Vestibular)
- Symptoms: Room spinning, nausea, hearing changes
- Exam: Nystagmus, positive head impulse test
- Think: Benign Paroxysmal Positional Vertigo (BPPV), vestibular neuritis, Meniere's
- Action: ENT referral, Epley maneuver for BPPV (**Fig. 19-2**)

CAUSE 2: Brain (Central)
- Symptoms: Imbalance + other neurologic signs
- Exam: Abnormal coordination tests, weakness, cognitive changes
- Think: Stroke, multiple sclerosis, cerebellar tumor
- Action: URGENT imaging and neurology

| FIGURE 23-1. CAUSES OF PROBLEMS WITH BALANCE AND COORDINATION |
|---|
| **Central Causes (Brain or Spinal Cord) of Balance and Coordination Problems**<br>Cerebellar Ataxia<br>Multiple Sclerosis<br>Parkinson's Disease<br>Stroke<br>Traumatic Brain Injury<br>Spinal Cord Injury (involvement of proprioceptive pathways)<br>Cerebral Palsy |
| **Peripheral Nervous System Causes of Balance and Coordination Problems**<br>Peripheral Neuropathy (loss of sensory feedback)<br>Guillain-Barré Syndrome |
| **Vestibular System Causes**<br>Vestibular Neuritis or Labyrinthitis<br>Benign Paroxysmal Positional Vertigo<br>Ménière's Disease<br>Central Vertigo |
| **Other Causes of Balance and Coordination problems**<br>Medication Side Effects<br>Alcohol, Drug Abuse, or Toxins<br>Muscular Weakness<br>Genetic Disorders, e.g., Friedreich's ataxia (ataxia, speech difficulty, muscle weakness), ataxia-telangiectasia (ataxia, speech difficulty, weakness, telangiectasia), Wilson's disease, Refsum's disease (buildup of phytanic acid can damage peripheral nerves, cerebellum, and vestibular system), and other hereditary ataxias)<br>Infections (e.g., encephalitis, inner ear infections)<br>Tumors (e.g., acoustic neuroma) |

CAUSE 3: Nerves/Sensation (Proprioceptive)

- Symptoms: Worse in dark, "walking on cotton"
- Exam: Loss of vibration/position sense
- Think: Diabetic neuropathy, B12 deficiency
- Action: Check A1c, B12, thyroid

Simple Bedside Test - Romberg:

- Stand with feet together, eyes closed for 30 seconds
- Normal: Slight sway but steady
- Abnormal: Falls or marked swaying = vestibular or proprioceptive problem

*Diagnosis of Balance and Coordination Problems*

**History**: Inquire about the time of onset, duration, progression, and specific circumstances under which these symptoms manifest. Review the patient's medications, possible exposure to potential neurotoxins, and familial history of neurological disorders.

**Physical Exam**: Assess mental status, blood pressure, cardiac rhythm, gait (ataxic gait, festinating gait [rapid short steps as in parkinsonism], or shuffling), stance (e.g., Romberg test), and coordination (e.g., finger-to-nose, heel-to-shin tests). Are there any cranial nerve deficits (CN 3, 4, 6 for eye movements, nystagmus); CN8 for vestibular and hearing sense)? Are there signs of muscle weakness, wasting or fasciculation? Are proprioception, vibration, and light touch intact? Are there any reflex abnormalities that might suggest a central or peripheral etiology?

**Imaging**: MRI of the brain and spinal cord is important in identifying structural lesions, demyelinating diseases, or cerebellar atrophies. CT scans may be utilized when MRI is contraindicated or in acute settings to rule out hemorrhagic conditions.

**Lab Tests**: Blood tests to identify metabolic disturbances, vitamin deficiencies (notably B12), thyroid dysfunction, or infectious causes.

**Specialized Tests**: Vestibular function tests, e.g., doll's eye test, videonystagmography, electronystagmography, rotary chair testing, posturography, vestibular evoked myogenic potentials (tests the muscular response to vestibular stimulation), hearing tests, nerve conduction studies, electromyography, or genetic testing (e.g., for Friedreich's ataxia or ataxia-telangiectasia) may be warranted based on initial findings.

***Treatment of Balance and Coordination Problems***

Depending on the cause:

**Physical and Vestibular Rehabilitation**: Exercises administered by a physical or occupational therapist to enhance balance, coordination, and muscle strength; helpful in peripheral vestibular disorders.

**Pharmacotherapy**:

- Vestibular suppressants, e.g., antihistamines (*meclizine [Antivert, Bonine], dimenhydrinate [Dramamine]), benzodiazepines (diazepam, lorazepam)* for vertigo
- Immunomodulatory agents for demyelinating diseases or specific treatments for Parkinson's disease

**Occupational Therapy**: Altering the patient's environment for safety

**Assistive Devices**: Canes, walkers, or wheelchairs, necessary for some patients

**Surgical Intervention**: Indicated in cases where structural lesions or vascular abnormalities are identified and amenable to surgical correction

Quick review of movement problems:

CEREBELLAR (Coordination Problems):

- Drunk-looking without alcohol
- Can't touch nose smoothly (intention tremor)
- Wide-based walking (ataxic gait)
- Slurred speech
- Think: Stroke, multiple sclerosis, alcohol, medications

BASAL GANGLIA (Unwanted Movements):

- Parkinson's: Slow, stiff, tremor at rest, shuffling walk
- Huntington's: Random jerky movements (chorea)
- Drug side effects: Weird movements from antipsychotic meds

Bottom Line:

- Clumsy / unsteady = cerebellum: Think stroke, alcohol, medications, multiple sclerosis.
- Weird movements = basal ganglia: Think Parkinson's or drug side effects

# 24

# *Changes in Vision*

Although a patient with changes in vision may see an ophthalmologist first, the neurologist may be called upon if there are other neurological symptoms.

Basic Patterns of Vision Loss:
SUDDEN VISION LOSS:

- One eye completely: Retinal artery occlusion, optic neuritis
- Same field both eyes: Stroke (homonymous hemianopia)
- Action: EMERGENCY ophthalmology + neurology

GRADUAL VISION LOSS:

- Central vision: Macular degeneration, cataracts
- Peripheral vision: Glaucoma, retinal detachment
- Action: Ophthalmology referral (urgent if retinal detachment)

DOUBLE VISION:

- One eye covered, still double: Eye problem (cataract, etc.)
- One eye covered, resolves: Nerve problem (CN 3,4,6)
- Action: Real double vision = Neurology referral

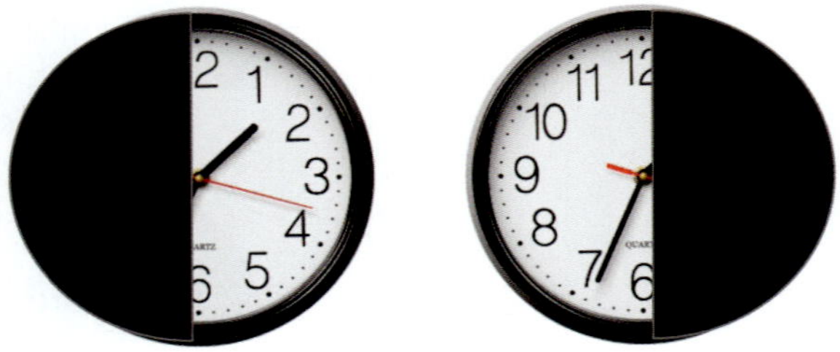


*Figure 24-1* *Bitemporal hemianopia with optic chiasm lesion.*

Non-neurological problems causing changes in vision are those affecting the cornea, uvea (iris, ciliary body, or choroid), lens, retina, or tear film. Neurological conditions include:

- Optic Neuritis (often associated with multiple sclerosis)
- Multiple Sclerosis (can cause other neurological problems involving the visual pathways due to demyelination)
- Stroke or Transient Ischemic Attack (when it affects the visual pathways)
- Migraine with Visual Aura
- Brain Tumors (which can occur near the optic nerve, chiasm, optic tract, or occipital or temporal lobe)
- Pituitary Adenoma (pressing on the optic chiasm, causing a bitemporal hemianopia; **Figs. 5-1** and **24-1**)
- Temporal Arteritis (can cause loss of vision in one or both eyes if the ophthalmic artery is involved)
- Cortical Blindness (can occur with damage to the occipital lobes, e.g., **Anton's syndrome**, where the patient is blind but denies it)
- Neurodegenerative Disease (Alzheimer's disease and Parkinson's disease may have problems with visual processing, including hallucinations.)
- Hereditary Optic Neuropathies, e.g., Leber's Hereditary Optic Neuropathy (sudden, painless central vision loss due to degeneration of retinal ganglion cells, of mitochondrial origin)
- Cranial Nerve Palsies (CNs 3, 4, 6)

***Diagnosis of Changes in Vision***

Diagnosing and treating changes in vision integrates both neurological and ophthalmological expertise. **History**: This includes the onset, duration, and progression of vision changes, associated symptoms (e.g., headache, weakness, seizures), systemic illnesses (e.g., diabetes, hypertension), and medication use.

**Physical Exam**: Check vision, using a near vision chart hand-held about 14 inches away (or a Snellen chart, viewed at 20 feet, if available), with the patient wearing her eyeglasses. Vision loss in only one eye points to pathology anterior to the optic chiasm, whether in the optic nerve or eye. If a lesion were posterior to the chiasm, it would affect vision in both eyes, since the visual pathways from both eyes merge posterior to the chiasm (**Fig. 5-1**). Assess for signs of decrease in mental status, motor weaknesses, sensory deficits, or alterations in reflexes. Give particular attention to cranial nerve function, especially the optic nerve (CN II), oculomotor (CN III), trochlear (CN IV), and abducens (CN VI) nerves for diplopia or nystagmus, as well as rough evaluation at least of the visual fields (**Fig. 12-1**). CN VI is one of most easily injured cranial nerves due to its long course. Examine the retina for papilledema (indicating increased intraocular pressure or papillitis). An ophthalmologist would include more formal visual fields, intraocular pressure, and slit-lamp examination.

**Imaging**:

- **MRI** of the brain and orbits with or without contrast enhancement to identify lesions affecting the visual pathways, such as tumors, demyelinating plaques, or strokes
- **CT Scan**: Useful in emergency settings, especially if intracranial hemorrhage or fractures are suspected

**Other Diagnostic Tests**:

**Visual Evoked Potentials (VEP)**: Used to assess the electrical activity in the visual pathway from the retina to the occipital cortex, and may be abnormal in multiple sclerosis, optic neuritis, or neuromyelitis optica (vision loss + spinal cord dysfunction)

**Fluorescein angiography** is used by ophthalmologists to visualize blood flow in the retina and choroid and can diagnose retinal diseases.

**Blood Tests**: To screen for systemic conditions, such as diabetes, hyperlipidemia, syphilis, or autoimmune disorders

*Treatment of Changes in Vision*

Ophthalmologic conditions will generally be managed by an ophthalmologist, such as anti-glaucoma medications, surgery for cataracts, prisms for diplopia, antibiotics for infections, surgical repair of retinal detachment, or intravitreal injections for macular degeneration.

For seizures or migraines with visual aura, appropriate antiepileptic or antimigraine medications may be prescribed by the neurologist. For multiple sclerosis, corticosteroids or disease-modifying therapies may be administered. In cases of stroke or transient ischemic attack, management may include antiplatelet drugs, statins, and control of risk factors (hypertension, diabetes).

**Rehabilitation** for patients with vision loss may include:

- Optical devices, such as magnifiers, telescopic glasses, video magnifiers, screen reading software, voice-activated devices, and computer apps for low vision users (e.g., converting text to speech)
- Instruction on the use of white canes, guide dogs, and other navigation means
- Training in skills at home for reading, cooking, and personal care
- Counseling and support
- Vocational counseling in finding employment, job training, and workplace accommodations
- Educational support using Braille and large print, and ways to access information

# 25

# Memory Loss and Cognitive Decline

Dementia is a broad term covering a range of neurological problems that affect cognitive function severely enough to interfere with daily life. It includes memory loss (especially short-term), reasoning ability (in planning or handling complex tasks or performing daily activities), communication (ability to find the right words in a conversation), disorientation (as to time, place, or identity of people), and changes in personality (e.g., irritability, depression, anxiety). *Dementia* differs from *delirium* in that dementia is a chronic progressive condition, while *delirium*, which commonly results from an acute illness or drug toxicity, is typically temporary, reversible over a few days to a few weeks.

Some degree of memory loss is a common part of aging. It is normal for older adults to:

- Forget names or appointments but remember them later
- Take longer to remember information; forget where they left their keys or why they just went into a particular room
- Have difficulty in multitasking

These difficulties, however, are mild and do not significantly impair daily functioning. They are part of the normal shrinkage of the brain with age. However, memory loss that disrupts daily life is not normal.

Symptoms that may raise a red flag are:

**Memory Loss Affecting Job Skills**: Forgetting things that are crucial to one's professional capabilities

**Difficulty Performing Familiar Tasks**: Struggling with tasks that were previously easy, such as managing finances or following recipes

**Language Problems**: Having trouble following or joining a conversation, or struggling to find the right words

**Disorientation**: Getting lost in familiar places or losing track of dates and seasons

**Poor Judgment**: Showing significant lapses in judgment or decision-making

**Misplacing Things**: Frequently placing items in unusual places and being unable to retrace steps to find them

**Mood and Personality Changes**: Experiencing mood swings, anxiety, irritability, or depression

Common causes of dementia include:

**Alzheimer's Disease**: The most common cause of dementia, characterized by the accumulation in the brain of *amyloid plaques* (beta-amyloid peptides, which collect outside the neurons) and *tau tangles* (tau proteins that accumulate inside the neuron), leading to the death of brain cells

**Vascular Dementia**: Caused by problems in the supply of blood to the brain, often due to strokes or atherosclerosis, leading to brain damage

**Lewy Body Dementia**: Associated with abnormal deposits in brain cells of alpha-synuclein protein (*Lewy bodies*). This can lead to problems with thinking, movement, behavior, and mood.

**Frontotemporal Dementia**: Results from abnormal accumulation of intercellular proteins and damage to the frontal and/or temporal lobes of the brain, which can affect behavior, personality, language, and movement. About one-third of cases have a familial tendency.

Less common causes of dementia include:

**Parkinson's Disease Dementia**: Develops in some people with Parkinson's disease

**Huntington's Disease**: A progressive brain disorder caused by a single autosomal dominant defective gene on chromosome 4. This defect causes changes in the central area of the brain (in men and women) that affect movement, mood, and cognitive abilities.

**Creutzfeldt-Jakob Disease (CJD)**: A rare, degenerative, fatal brain disorder caused by an abnormal infectious protein (a *prion*)

**Normal Pressure Hydrocephalus**: Caused by the buildup of fluid in the brain, which can lead to walking problems, urinary incontinence, and memory loss

**Wernicke-Korsakoff Syndrome**: A chronic memory disorder caused by severe deficiency of thiamine (vitamin B-1), most commonly caused by alcohol abuse

**Chronic Traumatic Encephalopathy**: Caused by repeated head trauma

**HIV-associated Dementia (HAD)**: Caused by infection of the brain by the human immunodeficiency virus (HIV)

**Mixed Dementia**: A condition in which changes representing more than one type of dementia occur simultaneously in the brain. For example, someone may have both Alzheimer's disease and vascular dementia.

*NOTE*: Some signs of dementia are reversible when caught early, e.g., those caused by nutritional deficiencies (vitamin B12, niacin, thiamine, vitamin D, omega-3 fatty acids, zinc), hyperthyroidism or hypothyroidism, autoimmune encephalopathy (e.g., Hashimoto's encephalopathy responds to steroids), infections (e.g., HIV, syphilis, Lyme disease), medication side effects, depression, normal pressure hydrocephalus, some brain tumors, alcohol abuse, hypoglycemia, hypercalcemia, subdural hematomas, sleep deprivation, and urinary tract infection (especially in the elderly).

For Acute Confusion (Hours to Days):

- Think: Delirium from infection, medications, metabolic
- Exam: Waxing / waning alertness or agitation (signs of delirium, not dementia, which is more chronic and progressive)
- Action: Check vitals, labs, medication list, treat underlying cause

For Gradual Memory Loss (Months to Years):

- Think: Dementia (Alzheimer's, vascular, etc.)
- Exam: Poor short-term memory, getting lost, personality changes
- Action: Cognitive testing, labs to rule out reversible cause

*Diagnosis of Dementia and Cognitive Loss*

**Figure 25-1** lists differences that can help differentiate the various kinds of dementia.

**Medical History**: Gather information about symptoms, family history of neurological diseases, and changes in behavior and personality.

**FIGURE 25-1. TYPES OF DEMENTIA**

| | Clinical Presentation | Neuroimaging | Biomarkers | Genetics |
|---|---|---|---|---|
| **Alzheimer's Disease** | Gradual onset with progressive memory loss and other cognitive impairments | MRI: Medial temporal lobe atrophy.<br>PET Scan: decreased metabolic activity in temporal and parietal lobes | • Decreased CSF amyloid-beta42<br>• Increased CSF tau and CSF phosphorylated tau | APOE epsilon4 allele |
| **Vascular Dementia** | Stepwise deterioration in cognitive function, often with a history of stroke or TIA | MRI: Evidence of cerebrovascular disease with infarcts, microbleeds, and loss of white matter volume | No specific markers | N/A |
| **Lewy Body Dementia** | • Fluctuating cognition, visual hallucinations, parkinsonism, loss of normal muscle relaxation during REM sleep.<br>• Cognitive decline may occur before or together with motor symptoms. | PET and SPECT scans may show decreased dopamine transporter uptake in the basal ganglia | Elevated CSF alpha-synuclein, tau, and phosphorylated tau protein | N/A |

| **Frontotemporal Dementia** | Changes in personality and behavior or language before memory loss | Frontal and/or temporal lobe atrophy on MRI | | Mutations in C9orf72, MAPT, and progranulin genes |
|---|---|---|---|---|
| **Parkinson's Disease Dementia** | Parkinsonism with later development of dementia | Similar findings as in Lewy Body Dementia | Similar to Lewy Body Dementia | |
| **Creutzfeldt-Jakob Disease** | • Rapidly progressing dementia, myoclonus, and ataxia<br>• EEG changes | MRI may show increased signal in the caudate and putamen on diffusion-weighted imaging. | • Elevated 14-3-3 protein in CSF<br>• Positive RT-QuIC assay for prion protein in CSF | |
| **HIV-Associated Dementia** | Subcortical (e.g., basal ganglia) dementia with motor symptoms, cognitive slowing, and behavioral changes | Atrophy and white matter changes in basal ganglia and frontal lobes with diffuse white matter changes on MRI | CSF may show increased HIV viral load | |
| **Wernicke-Korsakoff Syndrome** | • Persistent memory and cognitive effect.<br>• Anterograde and retrograde amnesia<br>• Confabulation<br>• Ophthalmoplegia, ataxia, and confusion<br>• May include nystagmus, hypothermia, hypotension, and coma when severe<br>• Thiamine deficiency | • MRI: Mammillary body atrophy; enhanced periaqueduct/third ventricle signal on T2/FLAIR images.<br>• Thalamic lesions, involvement of the cerebellum | • Low serum thiamine<br>• Liver enzymes may be elevated | May be a genetic predisposition affecting alcohol metabolism or nutritional absorption |
| **Chronic Traumatic Encephalopathy** | History of repetitive head trauma, with symptoms such as aggression, depression, impulsivity, and later cognitive decline | MRI may show atrophy, especially in the frontal and temporal lobes. | None | N/A |
| **Normal Pressure Hydrocephalus** | • Gait disturbances,<br>• Urinary incontinence<br>• Cognitive decline | • MRI or CT show enlarged ventricles.<br>• CSF pressure is normal. | | |

**Physical Exam**: Check for signs of stroke, Parkinson's disease, brain tumors, or other medical conditions that can affect brain function. Assess memory, problem-solving, attention, counting, and language skills. This can be done through the **Mini-Mental State Examination** or more formally through the **Montreal Cognitive Assessment** or through more comprehensive neuropsychological testing, e.g., the **Wechsler Adult Intelligence Scale**, the **California Verbal Learning Test**, or the **Trail Making Test**.

A Very Simple Memory Test:

- Orientation: Person, place, time, situation
- 3-word recall: Apple, penny, table (test after 5 minutes)
- Clock drawing: Draw clock showing 10 past 11 (screens for cognitive impairment by testing visuospatial skills, executive function, and working memory)

**Imaging**: MRI, CT, and PET scans can be used to examine brain structure and function changes.

**Lab Tests**: Blood tests (e.g., CBC, electrolytes, renal function tests, liver function tests, thyroid function tests, vitamin B12 and folate levels, calcium and glucose levels, HIV test, syphilis test [RPR or VDRL], CRP and ESR, toxicology screen, heavy metal screen) can help rule out other conditions that may cause similar symptoms.

**Psychiatric Evaluation**: To identify other conditions that could be causing or contributing to symptoms, such as depression

## Treatment of Dementia

**Medications**:

- For **Alzheimer's Disease**: **Cholinesterase inhibitors** (e.g., *donepezil, rivastigmine, galantamine)* to help manage memory, communication, and some behavioral problems by increasing the levels of acetylcholine. *Memantine* is used to treat moderate to severe Alzheimer's disease by blocking the excessive activation of glutamate receptors that leads to neuronal damage. *Lecanemab* (*Lequembi*) and *aducanumab* (*Aduhelm*) are monoclonal antibodies that targets and clear amyloid-beta plaques.
- **Antipsychotic medications** may be used to treat serious behavioral problems, but they come with significant risks, especially in older adults.
- For **Vascular Dementia**: Treatment for hypertension, hyperlipidemia, diabetes; antiplatelets for secondary stroke prevention. The focus is on cardiovascular health.
- For **Lewy Body Dementia**: Acetylcholinesterase inhibitors for cognitive symptoms; *carbidopa-levodopa* for parkinsonism; management of sleep disturbances; physical therapy
- For **Frontotemporal Dementia**: SSRIs or *trazodone* (a serotonin antagonist) for behavioral symptoms; speech therapy for language symptoms
- For **Parkinson's Disease Dementia**: Cholinesterase inhibitors for cognitive symptoms, dopaminergic therapy for motor symptoms; occupational therapy, physical therapy, speech therapy; atropine drops inside the mouth or botulinum toxin injection into the salivary glands for drooling
- For **Creutzfeldt-Jakob Disease**: No effective treatment except supportive care
- For **HIV-Associated Dementia**: Antiretroviral therapy, supportive care, cognitive rehabilitation, management of psychiatric symptoms

- For **Wernicke-Korsakoff Syndrome**: High-dose thiamine and management of alcohol abuse; nutritional support
- For **Chronic Traumatic Encephalopathy**: Symptomatic treatment for mood disorders, aggression, and cognitive impairment; behavioral therapy; cognitive therapy; support for families and caregivers
- For **Normal Pressure Hydrocephalus**: Treated with shunting, the most common being a ventriculoperitoneal shunt. Improvement of symptoms with shunting supports the diagnosis.

**Lifestyle Remedies**:
- **Regular exercise** can help improve mood and maintain the health of the heart, muscles, and joints.
- **Healthy diet** focusing on fruits, vegetables, whole grains, and lean protein can support brain health.
- **Cognitive stimulation** through puzzles, reading, and games

**Occupational therapy** can help with coping behaviors and strategies to make the environment safer.

**Speech therapy** can help with communication problems.

**Physical therapy** can assist with mobility and prevent falls.

**Support for Caregivers**: Providing education, support groups, and respite care options for caregivers is important, as caregiving can be very challenging.

**Advanced Care Planning**: Discuss and document care preferences, including end-of-life care and legal matters.

# 26

# Speech and Language Problems

**Aphasia** is difficulty with language production, comprehension, reading, or writing due to damage in the language-dominant (usually left) side of the brain. **Dysarthria** is slurred, slow speech, with muscle weakness and incoordination of the movements needed for speech but is otherwise linguistically normal. A number of neurological conditions can present with speech problems, either aphasia or dysarthria: stroke, neurodegenerative diseases (Alzheimer's disease and other dementias, primary progressive aphasia, Parkinson's disease, multiple system atrophy, progressive supranuclear palsy), amyotrophic lateral sclerosis, traumatic brain injury, brain tumors, epilepsy, multiple sclerosis, Huntington's disease, developmental disorders (autism spectrum disorders with specific language impairment), infectious and autoimmune diseases.

**Scanning speech** is a type of dysarthria with a peculiar staccato or halting rhythm, where the normal flow of speech is jerky, interrupted by irregular pauses and a variable rate of word production. It is typically associated with conditions affecting the cerebellum and is notable in multiple sclerosis.

*Diagnosis of Speech and Language Problems*

**History** should include the onset, progression, and pattern of the speech and language problems. Inquire whether there are associated symptoms such as weakness, cognitive changes, swallowing, or other difficulties, which might suggest a broader neurological condition.

**Neurological Exam:** Assess for signs of cognitive or focal neurologic deficits.

**Speech and Language Assessment:** A speech-language pathologist can help classify the type of speech or language disorder (e.g., aphasia, dysarthria), which is important for identifying the underlying neurologic condition.

In **motor aphasia (Broca's aphasia**), comprehension is preserved, but the patient has difficulty *finding* the right words and often speaks in short, broken phrases. Writing may also be affected.

The patient may be aware of and frustrated with, the problem. It is due to damage to Broca's area in the frontal lobe of the brain.

In **receptive aphasia (Wernicke's aphasia)**, the patient has difficulty *understanding* words. Speech may be fluent but nonsensical (a "word salad"), as the patient may hear but has difficulty understanding what he/she or others are saying. The patient may be unaware of the speech errors. Reading comprehension and writing are also impaired. It is due to damage to Wernicke's area in the superior temporal gyrus in the dominant hemisphere.

**Speech apraxia** is a problem with planning and coordinating the muscle movements needed for speech, without muscle weakness or loss of comprehension. The speech may be slow or hard to understand.

**Dysarthria** results from motor weakness or paralysis of speech muscles.

**Spasmodic dysphonia** is a chronic neurological voice disorder characterized by involuntary spasms during speech of the muscles that open or close the vocal cords, giving the voice a strained, strangled quality. Its exact cause is not clear, but may involve basal ganglia, cerebellar, or cerebral cortical dysfunction. It can be treated with speech therapy and botulinum toxin injection into the spasmodic muscles. Spasmodic dysphonia differs from the hoarseness and weak voice that come from vagus nerve injury, e.g., during neck surgery, that interrupts innervation to the vocal cords and may be treated with speech therapy.

**Imaging and Diagnostic Tests:** Based on the clinical findings, imaging studies such as MRI of the brain can identify structural abnormalities (e.g., stroke, tumor, degenerative changes). Additional tests like EEG, lumbar puncture, or blood tests may be indicated to rule out infection, inflammation, or metabolic conditions.

A quick assessment of aphasia vs dysarthria:

Dysarthria (Muscle Problem):

- Description: Slurred speech, sounds drunk
- Understanding: Normal (they know what they want to say)
- Causes: Stroke, Parkinson's, alcohol, medications
- Test: "Me-me-me" (lips - CN7), "La-la-la" (tongue - CN12), "Ga-ga-ga" (throat - CNs 9,10) - helps localize the source of the muscle problem

Aphasia (Brain Language Problem):

- Broca's (Motor): Understands but can't speak fluently
- Wernicke's (Sensory): Speaks fluently but doesn't make sense
- Causes: Left brain stroke, tumor
- Test: Ask to name objects, follow commands, repeat phrases

Quick Speech Assessment:

- Listen during history - obvious problems will be apparent
- Ask to repeat: "No ifs, ands, or buts" (if impaired, think motor aphasia or dysarthria)

- Ask to follow commands: "Close your eyes, stick out tongue" (if unable despite intact motor ability, suggests receptive aphasia or impaired attention)
- Ask to name: Point to common objects (if the patient cannot so so (e.g., pen, watch), this suggests anomia — a core feature of many aphasias (often Alzheimer's or stroke-related).

*Treatment of Aphasia*

Treatment should target the identified neurological condition. For example, in the case of stroke-induced aphasia, managing cardiovascular risk factors is important along with speech rehabilitation.

**Rehabilitation:** Speech and language therapy conducted by a speech-language pathologist is important for most speech and language disorders. The therapy focuses on improving communication abilities, compensatory strategies, and, where applicable, swallowing function.

**Medications:** While there are no specific medications for speech and language disorders, treating the underlying neurological condition (e.g., antiepileptics for seizures, immunomodulatory therapy for multiple sclerosis) can help alleviate symptoms.

**Surgical Intervention:** In rare cases, surgical treatment may be necessary, such as for removing a brain tumor causing speech and language problems.

**Supportive Care:** Cognitive rehabilitation, psychological support, and patient education about assistive communication devices or strategies can significantly improve the quality of life.

## Stuttering

Stuttering (stammering) is a speech disorder characterized by interruptions in normal speech flow, including repetitions, filler words (e.g., "like", "y'know"), prolongation of sounds, and speech blocks (inability to start a word), even though the stutterer may know exactly what he/she wants to say. It is often more pronounced under pressure or in certain social situations. Stuttering often begins in childhood and can disappear or continue into adulthood. The cause may include a combination of genetic, neurological and environmental factors.

*Diagnosis of Stuttering*

Assessment of stuttering is commonly conducted by a speech-language pathologist (SLP).

1. Case History: The SLP will ask about the individual's developmental, medical, and family history. Important aspects include:
   - Age of onset: When did stuttering begin?
   - Family history: Does stuttering run in the family?
   - Situational triggers: When is stuttering most severe? Does it worsen in social situations or under stress?
   - Associated factors: Any co-occurring conditions (e.g., anxiety, ADHD, or speech disorders).
2. Speech Assessment: Repetitions, prolongations, or blocks, and the conditions in which they occur (e.g., speaking alone versus in a group)

3. Severity: Standardized tools, such as the *Stuttering Severity Instrument (SSI)* test, may be used to quantify the severity of stuttering. The SLP may also assess the impact of stuttering on communication and quality of life.
4. Psychosocial Impact: Does the stuttering cause emotional distress, anxiety, or avoidance behaviors in social situations?

***Treatment of Stuttering***

Several treatment approaches can help reduce symptoms, depending on the person's age, the severity of the stuttering, and any related factors like anxiety or neurological conditions:

1. **Speech Therapy** is the most common and effective approach for managing stuttering:
   - *Fluency Shaping*: Focuses on teaching strategies to improve fluency, such as slow and controlled speech, gentle onset of speech, and breathing techniques.
   - *Stuttering Modification*: Helps individuals manage stuttering when it occurs, including easy stuttering and pull-out methods (stopping mid-stutter and easing out of it).
   - *Desensitization*: Involves gradually exposing individuals to speaking situations that trigger anxiety, helping them become more comfortable with their stutter.
2. **Cognitive-Behavioral Therapy (CBT)**: CBT can help individuals cope with the emotional aspects of stuttering, such as anxiety or negative self-perception. It focuses on changing negative thought patterns and reducing speech-related fears.
3. **Medications**: There presently are no FDA-approved medications specific for stuttering, but certain medications may help if stuttering is associated with anxiety or neurological conditions:
   - *Beta-blockers* or *anti-anxiety medications* can sometimes help with the anxiety that worsens stuttering in social situations, although they are not a cure for stuttering. *Guanfacine*, an ADHD drug, sometimes helps stuttering by lowering the levels of norepinephrine, leading to a calming effect with improved attention.
   - *Dopamine antagonists*: While first-generation antipsychotics (e.g., *haloperidol*) may help stuttering, they run the risk of significant side-effects (e.g., tardive dyskinesia). However, newer dopamine antagonists with a better side-effect profile (e.g., *ecopipam, deutetrabenazine*) are being tested.
   - *Anticonvulsants* (e.g., *gabapentin*): Occasionally used off-label to reduce neural hyperexcitability
4. **Assistive Devices**: Some individuals benefit from electronic devices that alter auditory feedback (e.g., delayed auditory feedback devices). These can help improve fluency by changing how the person hears their own voice.
5. **Support Groups**: Joining a support group or participating in online forums can provide emotional support and a sense of community for individuals who stutter.
6. **Self-help Approaches**: Practicing speech exercises can be useful. Mindfulness or relaxation techniques (e.g., deep breathing, progressive muscle relaxation) can help reduce the physical tension and anxiety associated with stuttering. Individuals may benefit from lowering pressure in speaking situations and focusing on communication rather than perfection.
7. **Treatment for Children**: For children, early intervention is important. Therapy focuses on developing smooth speech patterns, building confidence in speaking, and addressing any emotional concerns related to stuttering. Parents are often involved in the therapy process to help the child practice fluency techniques at home in a supportive environment.

# 27

# Changes in Mood or Behavior

*Diagnosis of Changes in Mood or Behavior*

**History:** What mood or behavior changes have been noted? When were they first noticed and how did they progress, suddenly or gradually? Do they include memory loss, motor problems, seizures, or any other changes? Is there a family history of a similar condition? Are there any situations, drugs, or medications that might have triggered the changes?

**Neurological Exam**: Note any neurologic findings that may suggest a particular lesion locus. Standardized tests for cognitive impairment and mood and behavioral changes may be useful, e.g., Mini-Mental State Examination test, Montreal Cognitive Assessment test.

**Neuropsychological Assessment**: Tests may include the Patient Health questionnaire, the Beck Depression Inventory, the Hamilton Depression Rating Scale, the Hamilton Anxiety Rating Scale, the Young Mania Rating Scale, the Frontal Assessment Battery.

**Imaging**: MRI and CT scans may identify structural brain abnormalities such as tumors, strokes, or evidence of neurodegenerative diseases. Functional imaging techniques, like PET and SPECT scans, can further delineate metabolic abnormalities and neuroinflammation.

**Lab Tests**: Blood tests can identify metabolic, genetic, and inflammatory conditions that may contribute to neurological and psychiatric symptoms. Specific tests may include thyroid function tests, vitamin B12 levels, autoimmune antibodies (lupus, Sjögren's syndrome), and cerebrospinal fluid analysis for infectious or inflammatory markers.

**EEG** can help if seizures or epilepsy are considered part of the differential diagnosis. EEG abnormalities can also correlate with the degree of an encephalopathy, as may be found in metabolic, hypoxic, infectious, or toxic encephalopathy.

| FIGURE 27-1. CAUSES OF CHANGES IN MOOD OR BEHAVIOR |
|---|
| Stroke |
| Traumatic Brain Injury |
| Aging |
| Hormonal Changes (e.g., during puberty, pregnancy, or menopause) |
| Brain Tumors |
| Epilepsy (especially before or after a seizure) |
| Multiple Sclerosis |
| Parkinson's Disease |
| Dementias (e.g., Alzheimer's disease) |
| Huntington's Disease |
| Encephalitis |
| Autoimmune Neurological Disorders (e.g., lupus, Sjögren's syndrome) |
| Neuroendocrine Disorders, e.g., Cushing's disease (cortisol effect), hypothyroidism |
| Neurosyphilis |
| Temporal Lobe Epilepsy |
| Wilson's Disease |
| Psychological (stress, trauma, grief, and other emotional conditions) |
| Medications (side effects of drugs, interactions between medications, or withdrawal from certain substances, such as drugs or alcohol) |
| Sleep Disturbances (lack of sleep or disruptions in sleep patterns) |
| Genetic Predisposition |
| Nutrition (diet and nutritional deficiencies can affect brain function and mood) |

*Treatment of Changes in Mood or Behavior*

**Medications:**

- **Antidepressants, mood stabilizers**, and **antipsychotic medications** can be employed to manage psychiatric symptoms based on the specific diagnosis and patient response.
- **Anti-epileptic drugs** may be indicated for mood stabilization and seizure control.
- **Disease-specific treatments** may be administered for specific neurological conditions (e.g., immunomodulatory therapies for multiple sclerosis, chelation for Wilson's disease, dopamine replacement for Parkinson's disease).

**Physical and occupational therapy** can improve functional outcomes and independence, particularly in conditions with motor impairment.

**Speech and language therapy** may be necessary for individuals with communication difficulties resulting from their neurological condition.

**Cognitive-behavioral therapy** by a mental health professional trained in cognitive-behavioral therapy can help develop coping strategies to manage mood disorders and behavioral changes.

# 28

# Sleep Disorders

Sleep plays a critical role in neurologic and general health. Disorders of sleep can lead to excessive daytime sleepiness, mood changes, cognitive decline, and even increased risk of stroke or cardiovascular disease. Sleep disorders may present first in neurologic disorders like Parkinson's disease or multiple sclerosis. Understanding the common sleep disorders—and knowing when to refer for a sleep study—is a key skill for the general clinician.

Sleep is divided into:

- Non-REM (NREM) sleep: Stages 1-3; deeper stages are restorative.
- REM (Rapid Eye Movement) sleep: Associated with dreaming and temporary muscle paralysis.

Sleep cycles through NREM and REM roughly every 90 minutes.

Sleep disorders can have many causes, including psychological, physical, environmental, or lifestyle factors (**Fig. 28-1**).

| FIGURE 28-1. CAUSES OF SLEEP DISORDERS |
|---|
| ***Psychological Factors*** |
| **Stress and Anxiety** |
| **Depression** (Too much or too little sleep are common symptoms of depression.) |
| **Bipolar Disorder**: Periods of high energy and depression can lead to significant sleep disturbances. |
| ***Physical Health Conditions*** |
| **Respiratory Disorders:** Conditions like asthma and chronic obstructive pulmonary disease (COPD) can disrupt sleep due to breathing difficulties. |
| **Neurological disorders** such as Parkinson's disease, Alzheimer's disease, and epilepsy can affect sleep patterns. |
| **Hormonal Imbalances** (E.g., hyperthyroidism can cause insomnia and other sleep disturbances.) |
| **Pain** (Chronic pain can make it difficult to fall asleep or stay asleep.) |
| **Gastroesophageal Reflux Disease (GERD)** can interrupt sleep. |
| **Sleep Apnea**: Obstructive sleep apnea, where breathing stops temporarily during sleep, significantly disrupts sleep. Obesity increases the risk of sleep apnea and other sleep-related breathing disorders. |
| **Restless Legs Syndrome** (an irresistible urge to move the legs) can prevent falling asleep. |
| **Narcolepsy**: A chronic sleep disorder characterized by overwhelming daytime drowsiness and sudden attacks of sleep. |
| **Pregnancy** (Hormonal changes, physical discomfort, and anxiety can affect sleep.) |
| **Genetic factors** can cause various sleep disorders involving changes in the circadian rhythm, insomnia, excessive sleepiness, or restless leg syndrome. |
| ***Environmental Factors*** |
| **Noise**: Loud or sudden noises can interrupt sleep. |
| **Light**: Exposure to light, especially blue light from screens, can interfere with melatonin production, affecting sleep. |
| **Temperature**: Extremes of temperature in the sleeping environment can prevent restful sleep. |
| ***Lifestyle Factors*** |
| **Irregular Sleep Schedule**: Shift work or frequent changes in sleep schedule can disrupt the body's circadian rhythm. |
| **Substance Use**: Alcohol, caffeine, and nicotine can affect sleep quality. Some prescription drugs can interfere with sleep as a side effect. |
| **Poor Sleep Hygiene**: Inadequate sleep environment (e.g., too bright, loud, or using screens before bed) and habits (e.g., eating heavy meals before bedtime) can lead to sleep disturbances. |

### *Diagnosis of Sleep Disorders*

**History:** What are the individual's sleep habits, including sleep patterns, duration, and quality (including snoring, gasping for breath, excessive daytime sleepiness, and leg discomfort at rest in tired patients)? Are there any stressors, medical conditions, medications, environmental or lifestyle factors that may be contributing to the sleep disturbance? A sleep diary can provide valuable information about sleep patterns and habits, including bedtime, wake time, total sleep time, and any disruptions or symptoms experienced during sleep.

**Sleep Questionnaires:** Various standardized questionnaires may be used to screen for specific sleep disorders or assess symptoms such as excessive daytime sleepiness, insomnia, restless legs syndrome, or sleep-related breathing disorders.

**Physical Exam:** For obesity, nasal congestion, enlarged tonsils, or other anatomical abnormalities

**Sleep Studies: Polysomnography (PSG)** and **home sleep apnea testing (HSAT)** are diagnostic tests used to evaluate sleep disorders such as obstructive sleep apnea, central sleep apnea (breathing pauses in sleep of CNS origin), periodic limb movement disorder (repetitive limb movements during sleep that disturb sleep continuity and may cause daytime sleepiness), and **parasomnias** (abnormal behaviors during sleep). PSG involves monitoring various physiological parameters during sleep, including brain activity, eye movements, muscle tone, heart rate, breathing patterns, and leg movements, and is typically conducted in a sleep laboratory. HSAT involves wearing a portable monitoring device at home to assess breathing patterns and oxygen levels during sleep.

Patients should be referred for polysomnography for:

- Loud snoring + daytime sleepiness (suspected obstructive sleep apnea)
- Sudden sleep attacks or cataplexy (suspected narcolepsy)
- Violent dream enactment (suspected sleep behavioral disorder)
- Unexplained nighttime events (parasomnias)

**Actigraphy:** A small device worn on the wrist measures movement. It can be useful in assessing insomnia and circadian rhythm disorders.

**MSLT (Multiple Sleep Latency Test):** Measures (in a sleep laboratory) how quickly a person falls asleep during the day. Used for narcolepsy.

**Psychological Assessment:** Where psychological factors, such as anxiety, depression, or post-traumatic stress disorder (PTSD) are suspected to contribute to sleep disturbances, a psychological evaluation may be recommended.

**Lab Tests:** Can assess for medical conditions that could be contributing to sleep disturbances, e.g., thyroid disorders, hormonal imbalances, or nutritional deficiencies

### *Treatment of Sleep Disorders*

Treatment of sleep disorders depends on the specific type.

**Sleep Hygiene Education:** This involves adopting healthy sleep habits and practices, such as maintaining a regular sleep schedule, creating a comfortable sleep environment, avoiding stimulants like caffeine and nicotine close to bedtime, and establishing a relaxing bedtime routine.

**Cognitive Behavioral Therapy for Insomnia (CBT-I):** CBT-I is a structured program that helps individuals address the thoughts and behaviors that contribute to insomnia.

It typically includes techniques such as cognitive restructuring, stimulus control, sleep restriction, and relaxation training.

**Medications:** Depending on the type and severity of the sleep disorder, medications may be prescribed such as benzodiazepines or non-benzodiazepine sedatives, as well as medications:

- For **restless legs syndrome**, dopamine agonists (e.g., *pramipexole* and *ropinirole*) may help reduce symptoms. Alpha-2 delta ligands (e.g., *gabapentin enacarbil* and *pregabalin*), typically used to treat epilepsy and neuropathic pain, may also be effective. Opioids like *oxycodone* or *tramadol* are generally reserved for cases that do not respond to other measures.
- For **narcolepsy**, stimulants (e.g., *modafinil*, *armodafinil*) help improve alertness and decrease daytime sleepiness. **Sodium oxybate**, by improving brain wave architecture, is effective in treating **cataplexy** (sudden loss of muscle tone and control triggered by strong emotions in some people with narcolepsy). Selective Serotonin Reuptake Inhibitors (SSRIs) and Serotonin-Norepinephrine Reuptake Inhibitors (SNRIs), e.g., *venlafaxine* or *fluoxetine*, are antidepressants that can help manage cataplexy and other symptoms of narcolepsy. *Pitolisant* (a brain histamine H3 receptor antagonist; brain histamine promotes wakefulness) or *solriamfetol* (a dopamine and norepinephrine reuptake inhibitor) are more recent options for treating narcolepsy.
- *Melatonin*, a naturally occurring sleep promoter, is useful for treating abnormalities involving circadian rhythm disturbances (e.g., jet lag, shift work sleep abnormalities, insomnia). In general, it is used to hasten the onset of sleep.
- Avoid chronic use of benzodiazepines or z-drugs (e.g., zolpidem) for insomnia, particularly in the elderly. These drugs may cause dependence; cognitive impairment; falls or other accidents; and adverse interactions with other drugs.

**Light Therapy:** Light therapy can be used to treat circadian rhythm disorders such as **delayed sleep-wake phase disorder** (persistent misalignment between a person's desired sleep-wake schedule and the person's internal biological clock) or **seasonal affective disorder** (depression that occurs seasonally during fall and winter months, associated with decreased exposure to sunlight). It involves exposure to bright artificial light, typically in the morning, to regulate the body's internal clock and improve sleep-wake patterns.

**Continuous Positive Airway Pressure (CPAP) Therapy:** CPAP is a common treatment for obstructive sleep apnea. It involves wearing a mask over the nose or mouth during sleep, which delivers a continuous stream of air to keep the airway open and prevent breathing pauses.

**Oral Appliances:** For individuals with mild to moderate obstructive sleep apnea or who cannot tolerate CPAP, oral appliances may be recommended. These are worn in the mouth during sleep to reposition the jaw and tongue, helping to keep the airway open.

**Treatment of Underlying Medical Conditions:** Addressing underlying medical conditions (such as depression, anxiety, chronic pain, or sleep-related movement disorders) can often improve sleep quality and reduce sleep disturbances.

**Lifestyle Modifications:** Making changes to lifestyle factors that can impact sleep (such as diet, exercise, and stress management) can also be beneficial in treating sleep disorders.

**Figure 28-2** reviews the diagnosis and treatment of common sleep disorders.

| FIGURE 28-2. DIAGNOSIS AND TREATMENT OF COMMON SLEEP DISORDERS | | | |
|---|---|---|---|
| **Disorder** | **Key Features** | **Diagnosis** | **First-Line Treatment** |
| **Obstructive Sleep Apnea (OSA)** | Snoring, gasping, daytime sleepiness. Associated with obesity, hypertension, and stroke risk. | Overnight **polysomnography** (PSG) | **CPAP** (Continuous Positive Airway Pressure), weight loss |
| **Insomnia** | Difficulty falling or staying asleep ≥3x/week for ≥3 months | Clinical | **Cognitive Behavioral Therapy for Insomnia (CBT-I)**; sleep hygiene |
| **Narcolepsy Type 1** | Excessive daytime sleepiness, **cataplexy** (sudden muscle weakness with emotion), sleep paralysis, hallucinations | PSG + **MSLT** (Multiple Sleep Latency Test) | **Modafinil** or **solriamfetol** for sleepiness; **sodium oxybate** for cataplexy |
| **Restless Legs Syndrome (RLS)** | Urge to move legs at rest, worse in evening | Clinical; check **ferritin** | Treat iron deficiency; **gabapentin** or **pramipexole** |
| **REM Sleep Behavior Disorder (RBD)** | Acting out dreams during REM sleep (loss of muscle paralysis) | PSG (shows REM without atonia) | Safety measures, **melatonin**, **clonazepam** |
| **Parasomnias** (e.g., sleepwalking, night terrors) | Occur during NREM sleep, usually in children | Clinical | Reassurance, safety precautions |

# 29

# Tumors of the Nervous System

Tumors of the nervous system can originate either inside the nervous system (primary) or outside the nervous system (metastatic) and can cause a great range of symptoms. Metastatic tumors are the most common brain tumors in adults (**Fig. 29-1**).

Classic Brain Tumor Triad (often not all present):

- Headache: New pattern, worse in morning, with vomiting
- Seizures: New onset, especially in adults >40
- Focal neurologic deficits: Weakness, speech problems, vision changes

Red-flag Headache Features:

- New headache in person >50 years old
- Headache that wakes you up
- Headache with nausea/vomiting (especially morning)
- Headache that's progressively worsening
- Headache, personality changes, or known cancer with neurologic symptoms

### *Diagnosis of Tumors of the Nervous System*

The neurologic exam helps to localize where the lesion is. Imaging tests help find the location and often can establish the fact that it is a tumor and what type it is. Frequently, though, biopsy is required to be sure of the exact pathology of the tumor, which may guide treatment.

### FIGURE 29-1. TUMORS OF THE NERVOUS SYSTEM

**PRIMARY BRAIN TUMORS**

**Gliomas** (arise from glial cells)

- *Astrocytomas*: Include low-grade, less aggressive, slower-growing astrocytomas, as well as high-grade, aggressive, faster-growing astrocytomas, like anaplastic astrocytomas and *glioblastoma multiforme*
- *Oligodendrogliomas*: Low or high grade, often affect the frontal and temporal lobes
- *Ependymomas*: Low- or high-grade, arise from ependymal cells that line the ventricular system
- *Brain Stem Gliomas*: Low- or high-grade, occur in the brain stem

**Meningiomas**: Arise from the meninges, typically benign but can be aggressive
**Pituitary Adenomas**: Benign tumors of the pituitary gland, which may be secreting or non-secreting
**Pineal Gland Tumors**: Include germinomas and pineoblastomas, both malignant
**Primary Central Nervous System (CNS) Lymphoma**: Malignant lymphoma that occurs in the brain
**Schwannomas**: Include vestibular schwannomas (acoustic neuromas), often benign. Although they arise from Schwann cells, which surround peripheral nerves, when they arise in the skull cavity, they can affect the brain or brain stem.
**Craniopharyngiomas**: Often benign tumors near the pituitary gland, arising from remnants of Rathke's embryonic pouch
**Medulloblastomas**: A type of primitive neuroectodermal malignant tumor (PNET), arising in the cerebellum and more common in children
**Gangliogliomas**: Rare, usually benign, tumors that contain both neuronal and glial elements
**Chordomas**: Malignant tumors that arise from remnants of the notochord, typically found at the base of the skull or the spine
**Hemangioblastomas**: Rare benign tumors that arise from blood vessels, often associated with Von Hippel-Lindau disease

**PRIMARY SPINAL TUMORS**

**Intradural-Intramedullary Tumors**: Such as astrocytomas and ependymomas *within* the spinal cord
**Intradural-Extramedullary Tumors**: Meningiomas and nerve sheath tumors like schwannomas and neurofibromas that occur within the dura and *outside* the spinal cord
**Extradural Tumors**: Typically involve metastases or originate from vertebral bones, such as chordomas, which are malignant

**PERIPHERAL NERVOUS SYSTEM TUMORS**

**Neurofibromas**: Typically benign, include solitary neurofibromas or those associated with neurofibromatosis
**Schwannomas**: Benign tumors of Schwann cells that can be associated with neurofibromatosis type 2
**Malignant Peripheral Nerve Sheath Tumors**: Cancerous growths that can arise from a neurofibroma

**METASTATIC BRAIN TUMORS**

Metastases to the brain can occur from lung, breast, melanoma, kidney, colorectal, and other cancers. Metastases are the most common brain tumors in adults.

**NOTE:** Even "benign" tumors can be very damaging by mass effect or, in the case of pituitary tumors, by excess hormone secretion.

*Treatment of Tumors of the Nervous System*

Treatment may consist of surgery, radiation, chemotherapy, targeted therapy (specifically targets cancer cells), immunotherapy (including steroids to reduce peritumor edema), non-invasive tumor treating field therapy (uses electric fields to disrupt cancer cell division and growth), or palliative care, depending on the type of tumor, its location, and the condition of the patient for undergoing surgery.

# Glossary

*acoustic neuroma*—a tumor of the Schwann cell elements of the auditory nerve
*anesthesia*—absence of sensation
*anterograde amnesia*—inability to form new memories after the causative event
ADHD—Attention Deficit Hyperactivity Disorder
*aneurysm*—a focal ballooning out of a segment of blood vessel wall
*anhidrosis*—decreased sweating
*Babinski reflex*—an abnormal reflex in which the great toe moves upward and the toes fan upon stroking the lateral plantar surface of the foot. It generally signifies an upper motor neuron lesion in an adult but is normal in an infant.
*basal ganglia*—caudate nucleus, lentiform nucleus (= putamen plus globus pallidus), claustrum and amygdala
*bilateral*—both sides of the body
*bitemporal hemianopia*—loss of the temporal (lateral) visual field in each eye
*brachial artery*—the major artery to the upper extremity, arising from the subclavian artery
*bradykinesia* – slowness of movement
*Brodmann's areas*—a classification of areas of the cerebral cortex according to assigned numbers
*calcarine fissure*—the horizontal fissure on the medial aspect of the occipital lobe. It separates the projections from the superior retinae (above) and the inferior retinae (below).
*cauda equina*—the bundle of nerve roots extending caudally from the caudal end of the spinal cord
*cerebral cortex*—the narrow zone of gray matter that lies at the surface of the cerebrum. The gray matter lies external to the white matter in the cerebrum. The reverse is true for the spinal cord
*circumlocution*—the use of many words to express what might be stated by few or one
*coma*—depressed consciousness to the degree of unresponsiveness to noxious stimuli
*conductive hearing loss*—hearing deficit resulting from a mechanical defect in the transmission of sound information between the external ear and the neuronal sensory apparatus (as opposed to neuronal hearing loss)
*confabulation*—production of fabricated memories which the subject often believes to be true
*conjugate gaze*—symmetrical movements of the eyes in a given direction
*contralateral*—the opposite side of the body
*converge*—to move (the eyes) toward one another
*corpus callosum*—the major connecting pathway between left and right hemispheres
*corticobulbar tract*—the motor pathway between the motor area of the cerebral cortex and the brain stem nuclei
*deja vu phenomenon*—the feeling of having previously experienced a current event
*diencephalon*—thalamus, hypothalamus, epithalamus, plus subthalamus
*dermatome*—the area of skin supplied by one nerve root
*dilation*—expansion
*diplopia*—double vision

*fasciculations*—coarse muscle twitching seen with peripheral motor nerve injury
*fibrillations*—fine, rarely visible, twitching of single muscle fibers, seen with peripheral motor nerve injury
*flaccid paralysis*—paralysis in which the affected muscles are limp, with little resistance to passive movement
*gastroparesis*—delayed emptying of the stomach
*hemiplegia*—paralysis of the extremities on one side of the body
*homonymous hemianopia*—loss of half of the visual field in each eye for a given side of the environment
*homunculus*—the upside-down representation of the human body on the cerebral cortex
*Horner's syndrome*—pupillary constriction, slight ptosis, and decreased sweating resulting from interruption of the sympathetic pathways to the eye (ptosis, miosis, and anhidrosis)
*hyperpyrexia*—elevation of body temperature
*hyperreflexia*—overactive reflexes
*hyporeflexia*—underactive reflexes
*Idiopathic*—of unknown origin
*infarction*—a region of tissue death, resulting from obstruction of the local circulation
*intercostal arteries*—the arteries that run between the ribs. These give contributory branches to the spinal cord
*intermediolateral columns*—the autonomic zone of spinal cord gray matter, which lies between the anterior and posterior gray horns
*interpalpebral fissure*—the space between the upper and lower eyelids
*intrathecal*—in the subarachnoid space around the spinal cord
*ipsilateral*—the same side of the body
*lamina terminalis*—an emotion-related pathway connecting amygdala with hypothalamus
*lesion*—injury
*lethargy*—drowsiness
*medially*—toward the midline
*meninges*—the outer lining of the central nervous system (pia, arachnoid, and dura)
*meningitis*—inflammation of the meninges
*mesencephalic nucleus of 5*—the rostral-most part of the sensory nucleus of CN5
*miosis*—constriction of the pupil
*nasolabial fold*—the skin crease extending from the nose to a point lateral to the corner of the mouth
*neologism*—the use of a new word or an old word in a new sense
*neuron*—nerve cell
*neuronal hearing loss*—hearing deficit resulting from damage to CN8
*obex*—the caudal-most landmark of the fourth ventricle
*obtundation, stupor*—progressive degrees of depressed consciousness between lethargy and coma
*olfaction*—the sense of smell
*olive*—the inferior olivary nucleus in the medulla
*ossicles*—the small ear bones that transmit sound
*papilledema*—swelling of the optic nerve head
*papillitis*—inflammation of the optic nerve head
*paresis*—partial weakness, short of paralysis (which is total)

*periaqueductal gray*—the gray matter around the aqueduct, containing high concentrations of endorphins, which are opioid peptides
*posterior columns*—the fasciculus gracilis plus fasciculus cuneatus
*pretectum*—the area just deep to the superficial regions of the superior colliculus
*proprioception*—the ability to sense the position of the limbs and their movements, with the eyes closed
*ptosis*—drooping of the eyelid
*pyramidal decussation*—crossover site of the corticospinal tracts
*radicular pain*—pain along the distribution of a nerve root or primary nerve trunk
*reflex*—an involuntary motion resulting from a stimulus (e.g. biceps jerk in response to percussion of the biceps tendon)
*retina*—the light-sensitive neural membrane within the eye
*retrograde*—in reverse direction
*retrograde amnesia*—loss of memories formed before the causative event
*sagittal*—in a plane parallel to that which divides an animal into right and left halves
*septum pellucidum*—the thin midline membrane, between right and left lateral ventricles
*spastic paralysis*—paralysis with a coinciding steady and prolonged involuntary contraction of the muscles
*stereognosis*—the ability to recognize objects by touching and handling them with the eyes closed
*stria medullaris*—a limbic system pathway on the dorsomedial surface of the thalamus, connecting septal to habenular nuclei
*stroke*—a prolonged or permanent loss of function in a brain area, resulting from interruption of the blood supply
*subthalamus*—a nuclear region just lateral to the hypothalamus; lesions may result in hemiballismus (violent, flailing movements of a limb)
*tardive dyskinesia*—involuntary, repetitive movements, typically of the face, lips, tongue, and limbs, often caused by long-term use of certain antipsychotic medications, particularly dopamine antagonists
*telangiectasia*—spidery dilation of small blood vessels near the skin surface
*tympanic membrane*—the vibratory membrane separating the external and middle ear
*uncus*—a portion of the temporal lobe concerned with the sense of smell. Epileptic seizures in this area are characterized by unpleasant smells. The uncus lies close to CN3 and may press upon and injure it following a subdural hemorrhage that forces the uncus to herniate against the brain stem.
*unilateral*—on one side
*vestibular apparatus*—the balance-sensing mechanism in the inner ear
*visual field*—the portion of the environment that the eye(s) sees on fixed forward gaze

# Index

*RAPID LEARNING AND RETENTION THROUGH THE MEDMASTER SERIES:*

*BASIC SCIENCES:*

**CLINICAL NEUROANATOMY MADE RIDICULOUSLY SIMPLE,** by S. Goldberg
**CLINICAL BIOCHEMISTRY MADE RIDICULOUSLY SIMPLE,** by S. Goldberg
**ORGANIC CHEMISTRY MADE RIDICULOUSLY SIMPLE,** by G.A. Davis
**CLINICAL ANATOMY MADE RIDICULOUSLY SIMPLE,** by S. Goldberg and H. Ouellette
**CLINICAL PHYSIOLOGY MADE RIDICULOUSLY SIMPLE,** by S. Goldberg
**CLINICAL MICROBIOLOGY MADE RIDICULOUSLY SIMPLE,** by M.T. Gladwin, B. Trattler and C.S. Mahan
**CLINICAL PHARMACOLOGY MADE RIDICULOUSLY SIMPLE,** by J.M. Olson
**ACID-BASE, FLUIDS, AND ELECTROLYTES MADE RIDICULOUSLY SIMPLE,** by R. Preston
**PATHOLOGY MADE RIDICULOUSLY SIMPLE,** by A. Zaher
**CLINICAL PATHOPHYSIOLOGY MADE RIDICULOUSLY SIMPLE,** by A. Berkowitz
**CLINICAL BIOSTATISTICS AND EPIDEMIOLOGY MADE RIDICULOUSLY SIMPLE,** by A. Weaver and S. Goldberg
**HOW CONSCIOUSNESS ARISES: A New Theory of Mind in Humans, Nature, and Machines,** by S. Goldberg
**CLINICAL GENETICS MADE RIDICULOUSLY SIMPLE,** by S. Goldberg

*CLINICAL SCIENCES:*

**OPHTHALMOLOGY MADE RIDICULOUSLY SIMPLE,** by S. Goldberg and W. Trattler
**PSYCHIATRY MADE RIDICULOUSLY SIMPLE,** by J. Nelson, W. Good and M. Ascher
**CLINICAL PSYCHOPHARMACOLOGY MADE RIDICULOUSLY SIMPLE,** by J. Preston and J. Johnson
**BEHAVIORAL MEDICINE MADE RIDICULOUSLY SIMPLE,** by F. Seitz and J. Carr
**THE FOUR-MINUTE NEUROLOGIC EXAM,** by S. Goldberg
**CLINICAL RADIOLOGY MADE RIDICULOUSLY SIMPLE,** by H. Ouellette and P. Tetreault
**THE PRACTITIONER'S POCKET PAL: ULTRA RAPID MEDICAL REFERENCE,** by J. Hancock
**CLINICAL CARDIOLOGY MADE RIDICULOUSLY SIMPLE,** by M.A. Chizner
**CARDIAC DRUGS MADE RIDICULOUSLY SIMPLE,** by M.A. Chizner and R.E. Chizner
**CARDIAC PHYSICAL EXAM MADE RIDICULOUSLY SIMPLE,** by M.A. Chizner
**ECG INTERPRETATION MADE RIDICULOUSLY SIMPLE,** by M.A. Chizner
**ORTHOPEDICS MADE RIDICULOUSLY SIMPLE,** by P. Tétreault and H. Ouellette
**IMMUNOLOGY MADE RIDICULOUSLY SIMPLE,** by M. Mahmoudi
**ALLERGY AND ASTHMA MADE RIDICULOUSLY SIMPLE,** by M. Mahmoudi
**RHEUMATOLOGY MADE RIDICULOUSLY SIMPLE,** by A.J. Brown
**CRITICAL CARE AND HOSPITALIST MEDICINE MADE RIDICULOUSLY SIMPLE,** by M. Donahoe and M.T. Gladwin
**CLINICAL HEMATOLOGY MADE RIDICULOUSLY SIMPLE,** by S. Goldberg
**ARE YOU AFRAID OF SNAKES?: A Doctor's Exploration of Alternative Medicine,** by C.S. Mahan
**WAR AGAINST THE GERMS: EPIDEMICS, MICROORGANISMS, AND BIOWARFARE,** by S. Goldberg
**ENDOCRINOLOGY MADE RIDICULOUSLY SIMPLE,** by S. Goldberg
**GASTROENTEROLOGY MADE RIDICULOUSLY SIMPLE,** by S. Goldberg
**NEUROLOGY MADE RIDICULOUSLY SIMPLE,** by S. Goldberg and D. Salzman
**ROUTINE LAB VALUES MADE RIDICULOUSLY SIMPLE,** by S. Goldberg

*BOARD REVIEW:*

**USMLE STEP 1 MADE RIDICULOUSLY SIMPLE,** by A. Carl
**USMLE STEP 2 MADE RIDICULOUSLY SIMPLE,** by A. Carl
**USMLE STEP 3 MADE RIDICULOUSLY SIMPLE,** by A. Carl
**NCLEX-RN MADE RIDICULOUSLY SIMPLE,** by A. Carl

*OTHER:*

**MEDICAL SPANISH MADE RIDICULOUSLY SIMPLE,** by T. Espinoza-Abrams
**MED SCHOOL MADE RIDICULOUSLY SIMPLE,** by S. Goldberg
**MED'TOONS** (260 humorous medical cartoons by the author) by S. Goldberg
**THE STUTTERER'S APPRENTICE,** by A. Splaver

For further information, see http://www.medmaster.net or Email: info@medmaster.net.